ESSENTIALS OF ASPIRATION BIOPSY CYTOLOGY

ESSENTIALS OF ASPIRATION BIOPSY CYTOLOGY

GIA-KHANH NGUYEN, M.D.
Pathologist
University of Alberta Hospitals
And
Associate Professor of Pathology
Faculty of Medicine
University of Alberta
Edmonton, Alberta, Canada

TILDE S. KLINE, M.D.
Associate Pathologist
Chief, Division of Cytology
Lankenau Hospital
And
Professor of Pathology
Thomas Jefferson Medical School
Philadelphia, Pennsylvania

IGAKU-SHOIN 1944

Igaku-Shoin New York · Tokyo

Published and distributed by

IGAKU-SHOIN Medical Publishers, Inc.
1140 Avenue of the Americas, New York, N.Y. 10036

IGAKU-SHOIN Ltd.,
5-24-3 Hongo, Bunkyo-ku, Tokyo

Library of Congress Cataloging-in-Publication Data

Nguyen, Gia-Khanh.
Essentials of aspiration biopsy cytology / by Gia-Khanh Nguyen, Tilde S. Kline.
p. cm.
Includes bibliographical references.
Includes index.
1. Cancer—Cytodiagnosis. 2. Biopsy, Needle. I. Kline, Tilde S. II. Title.
[DNLM: 1. Biopsy, Needle. 2. Cytodiagnosis. 3. Diagnosis, Differential. 4. Neoplasms—diagnosis. QZ 241 N576e]
RC270.3.C97N48 1991
616.99'407582—dc20
DNLM/DLC
for Library of Congress 90-5005
CIP

ISBN: 0-89640-188-X (New York)
ISBN: 4-260-14188-0 (Tokyo)

Printed and bound in the U.S.A.

10 9 8 7 6 5 4 3 2 1

Acknowledgment

We wish to acknowledge Ms. Lynda Harrison and Mr. Dick Golda of the Department of Pathology, University of Alberta, and Ms. Michelle Darby of the Department of Pathology, Lankenau Hospital for their valuable help in the preparation of the manuscript. Last, but not least, we thank Ms. Lila Glass Maron, Mr. David Lasky, and the production staff of Igaku-Shoin, New York for their technical expertise, valued suggestions, and enthusiasm in publishing our work.

Gia-Khanh Nguyen, M.D.
Tilde S. *Kline*, M.D.

Preface

Essentials of Aspiration Biopsy Cytology is the result of our experience gained from many years of active involvement in teaching cytology to residents and fellows in pathology and cytotechnology students. Information has also been gathered from presentations made by the authors at several cytology workshops at local, regional, and national professional meetings. The book is specifically written for practicing pathologists in community hospitals, pathology residents, and cytotechnologists. It has fourteen chapters containing basic information that one needs to know for a safe and accurate diagnostic aspiration biopsy cytology. Almost all major lesions investigated by needle aspiration biopsy are described and illustrated. Only exceedingly rare tumors and tumor-like lesions are intentionally omitted. The practical value and limitations of cytochemistry, immunocytochemistry and electron microscopy in tumor typing are briefly discussed; cytologic differential diagnoses and diagnostic traps are emphasized. Specialists in other medical specialties who are interested in needle aspiration biopsy and candidates for specialty board examinations will find this concise book informative.

Gia-Khanh Nguyen, M.D.
Tilde S. Kline, M.D.

Contents

1. **INTRODUCTION 1**
   History 1
   Utilization 2
   Safety 2
   Diagnostic Criteria 2
   Pitfalls of Diagnosis 3
   The Report 4
   Caveat 4
   Philosophy 4

2. **CLINICAL AND LABORATORY PROCEDURES 7**
   Biopsy Procedure 7
   Equipment 7
   Biopsy Technique 8
   Complications 9
   Transthoracic NAB 10
   Transabdominal NAB 10
   Preparation of Specimens 10
   Direct Smear 10
   Cytocentrifuge Smear 10
   Membrane Filtrate 11
   Cell Block 11
   Electron Microscopic Study 11
   Routine Staining Methods 11
   Immunocytochemical Staining Methods 12

3. BREAST 14

Indications and Contraindications for NAB 14

Benign Nonneoplastic Lesions 14

Inflammatory Disorders 14

Fibrocystic Changes 15

Benign Tumors 18

Malignant Tumors 20

Ductal Carcinoma 20

Common Ductal Carcinoma Variants 20

Lobular Carcinoma 23

Other Breast Cancers 26

Diagnostic Accuracy and Pitfalls 26

4. THYROID AND PARATHYROID 27

Thyroid 27

Indications and Contraindications for NAB 27

Normal Thyroid 27

Thyroid Cysts 28

Thyroiditis 28

Hyperplasia 30

Neoplasms 31

Diagnostic Accuracy 38

Diagnostic Pitfalls 40

Parathyroid 41

5. SALIVARY GLANDS AND OTHER NECK MASSES 43

Indications and Contraindications for NAB 43

Salivary Glands 44

Benign Nonneoplastic Lesions 44

Benign Tumors 45

Malignant Tumors 47

Branchial Cleft Cyst 50

Carotid Body Tumor 50

Diagnostic Accuracy 51

Diagnostic Pitfalls 51

6. LYMPH NODES 54

Indications and Contraindications for NAB 54

Lymphadenitis 55

Lymphoma 56

Hodgkin's Lymphoma 56
Non-Hodgkin's Lymphoma 56
Metastatic Cancer 57
Squamous Cell Carcinoma 60
Adenocarcinoma 60
Transitional Cell Carcinoma 63
Anaplastic Carcinoma 63
Neuroendocrine Tumor 64
Germ Cell Tumor 64
Melanoma 67
Diagnostic Accuracy 67
Diagnostic Pitfalls 69

7. BONE AND SOFT TISSUE 72
Bone 72
Indications for NAB 72
Primary Bone Tumors 73
Metastatic Cancers 75
Diagnostic Accuracy and Pitfalls 77
Soft Tissue 77
Indications for NAB 77
Lipomatous Tumors 77
Spindle-Cell Tumors 79
Pleomorphic Tumors 81
Round-Cell Tumors 82
Metastatic Cancer 85
Diagnostic Accuracy and Pitfalls 85

8. PROSTATE 88
Indications and Contraindications for NAB 88
Benign Prostatic Enlargement 89
Prostatitis 89
Carcinoma 90
Cellular Changes Due to Hormonal Therapy 94
Diagnostic Accuracy and Pitfalls 94

9. LUNG, PLEURA AND MEDIASTINUM 97
Indications and Contraindications for NAB 97
Normal Lung 98
Inflammatory Lung Lesions 99

Hamartoma 102
Malignant Tumors of the Lung 105
Bronchogenic Carcinoma 105
Carcinoid Tumor 111
Other Lung Cancers 111
Diagnostic Accuracy and Pitfalls 112
Tumors of the Pleura 113
Mediastinal Space-Occupying Lesions 114

10. PANCREAS AND AMPULLARY REGION 117
Indications and Contraindications for NAB 117
Normal Pancreas 118
Inflammatory Lesions 119
Pancreatic Cystic Lesions 120
Carcinoma of Duct Cell Origin 121
Metastatic Cancer 123
Ampullary Carcinoma 123
Neuroendocrine Tumor 124
Diagnostic Accuracy 124
Diagnostic Pitfalls 125

11. LIVER, GALLBLADDER, AND BILE DUCTS 127
Indications and Contraindications for NAB 127
Liver 128
Normal Liver 128
Benign Hepatic Lesions 129
Hepatocellular Carcinoma 131
Cholangiocarcinoma 134
Metastatic Cancer 135
Neoplasms of the Gallbladder and Extrahepatic Bile Ducts 136
Diagnostic Accuracy and Pitfalls 138

12. KIDNEY AND ADRENAL 139
Indications and Contraindications for NAB 139
Kidney 140
Normal Kidney 140
Benign Renal Mass Lesions 140
Malignant Renal Tumors 142
Carcinomas of the Renal Pelvis 144
Adrenal 146

Tumors of the Cortex 146
Tumors of the Medulla 146
Metastatic Cancer 149
Diagnostic Accuracy and Pitfalls 151

13. CENTRAL NERVOUS SYSTEM 152
Indications and Contraindications for NAB 153
Normal Cerebrum 153
Reactive Gliosis 153
Tumors of the Cerebrum and Cerebellum 156
Neuroectodermal Tumors 156
Metastatic Cancer 158
Pituitary Adenoma 159
Meningioma 161
Acoustic Neuroma or Neurilemoma 161
Diagnostic Accuracy and Pitfalls 163

14. DNA QUANTITATION 165
Cell Cycle 165
DNA Quantitation Methods 166

15. APPENDIX 170
Questions 170

INDEX 179

KEYS TO ABBREVIATIONS

ABC	Aspiration Biopsy Cytology
NAB	Needle Aspiration Biopsy

1

INTRODUCTION

HISTORY

Aspiration biopsy cytology (ABC) is not a recent innovation. Since the mid-19th century, reports of aspirated specimens have described the findings not only of tumor cells but also of specific microorganisms. The trio regarded as the fathers of aspiration biopsy cytology, however, are the clinician, Hayes Martin; the technologist, Edward Ellis; and the pathologist, Fred Stewart. In 1930 at New York's Memorial Hospital these men, by means of a cooperative venture, the team approach, issued a report of 65 cases procured from multiple body sites. This article and a subsequent one from 1933 based on more than 700 biopsies aroused little interest in the United States, where both pathologist and clinician preferred the customary excisional biopsy. In war-torn Europe, however, needle aspiration biopsy (NAB) had an impressive following. In 1954, Paul Lopes Cardozo from the Netherlands published two volumes on this procedure. In socialized Sweden in 1966 the clinician Nils Söderström wrote a provocative text on the general subject, while Sven Dahlgren and Björn Nordenström provided a monograph on radiographically-assisted aspiration biopsies from pulmonary lesions. Thereafter, out of Radiumhemmet came a wealth of material. By the late 1960s in the United States interest had focused on NAB from pulmonary lesions, and at Lankenau Hospital in 1970, the procedure was applied to lesions of the breast. With increasing governmental regulations and restrictions and spiraling costs connected with hospitalization, this mode of examination became an accepted technique. Now, at the commencement of the final decade of the 20th century, it is an established biopsy procedure involving residents, pathologists, and clinicians. The American Board of Pathology, recognizing the role of ABC in anatomic pathology, has increased the emphasis on its interpretation in the Anatomic Boards and in 1989 administered the first "added qualification" examination in cytopathology.

UTILIZATION

Targeted for examination by the NAB technique is the gamut of tissue from all areas of the body. These lesions may be visible, palpable, or deep masses viewed by imaging modalities.

The principle aim of NAB is distinction of the malignant lesion from the benign one and definitive diagnosis. It can be used successfully in the realm of microbiology, as well. A number of special studies, such as immunocytochemistry and electron microscopy, can also be applied to the aspirated specimen—allying it even more closely to excisional biopsy. Finally, prognostication, based on utilization of the aspirated specimen through such tools as image analysis and flow cytometry, is becoming a reality.

SAFETY

The major deterrent to acceptability of the procedure has been the fear that NAB would seed tumor cells. This erroneous concept, eagerly embraced by reluctant clinicians, is almost a myth. Amid thousands of reports related to aspiration biopsy, only a handful of cases (almost entirely limited to patients with carcinomatosis) have shown this dreaded complication, and among these patients the procedure had obviated hospitalization and extensive unnecessary surgery. Other complications cited include hemorrhage and infection. The former is rarely a problem with the 22-gauge needle, even in patients with clotting defects, and the latter is also unusual.

DIAGNOSTIC CRITERIA

The criteria of malignancy of ABC differ in part from those of exfoliative cytology. In the former, examination is based, in part, on the pattern of the cells, whereas in the latter, it is based on the features of the individual cell. The major ABC criteria of malignancy are:

Cellularity
Dyshesion
Monomorphism
Nuclear irregularity
Anisonucleosis
Macronucleoli

The pattern approach to ABC constitutes preliminary evaluation of the specimen. With the scanning or low-power objective lens, the slide is examined for cellularity, dyshesion (loss of intercellular cohesion), and monomorphism (a single type of epithelium). By means of this initial examination, both a tentative and a differential diagnosis are made. Thereafter, with the high-power objective lens the cells are evaluated for nuclear membrane irregularity and thickening, anisonucleosis (variable sizes), and macronucleoli. Nuclear/cytoplasmic ratio alteration and chromatin clumping are not salient criteria for assessment of ABC, by contrast to assessment of exfoliative cytology. The significance of background substance, or "tumor diathesis," is chiefly to distinguish an inflammatory from a noninflammatory process and to recognize diagnostic material, such as colloid or mucin.

Every tumor from each site obviously does not display all the major characteristics of malignancy. Similarly, use of criteria for evaluation of exfoliative cytology is selective, e.g., cells from squamous carcinoma reveal prominent alteration in nuclear/cytoplasmic ratio and chromatin detail by contrast to those from endometrial adenocarcinoma, wherein anisonucleosis and macronucleoli are paramount. Moreover, some of the ABC criteria of malignancy are associated with certain benign lesions. For example, the specimen from a benign fibroadenoma of the breast frequently is cell-rich, as are all satisfactory specimens from lymph nodes. Nevertheless, inspection of aspirates for all major malignant criteria is a vital approach and should be applied as the first step to interpretation of samples from all organs.

The criteria of benignity contrast with those of malignancy and include:

- Cell sparsity
- Cohesion
- Polymorphism
- Polarized equal-sized nuclei
- Cytoplasmic membrane delineation
- Cytoplasmic secretions and inclusions

Evaluation of the sample for cell numbers often is the prime indicator regarding the nature of the lesion. Cell sparsity, however, can be a problem. What is the critical number of epithelial cells for a representative, yet adequate, benign specimen? For mammary and prostatic lesions, we suggest that three to six epithelial cell groups per slide generally constitute a satisfactory sample, particularly when taken by the experienced hand.

PITFALLS OF DIAGNOSIS

Although each organ has certain special diagnostic pitfalls, a number are common to all. Awareness often means avoidance of the majority. False-negatives generally result from three traps: fibrosis or desmoplasia, incarcerating the tumor cells; well-differentiated tumor cells, mimicking normal cells; and the geographic miss secondary to inexperience, tumor size, or location. A false-positive diagnosis may be made because of pregnancy, which stimulates cellularity, anisonucleosis, and the appearance of eosinophilic macronucleoli; contamination, particularly in conjunction with lesions sampled with the aid of imaging modalities; and heterotopia, since "alien cells" from lymphadenopathy are an indication of metastatic tumor. Both false-positives and false-negatives may be secondary to the changes caused by inflammatory conditions, radiation, and chemotherapy.

These snares often can be evaded by discriminating use of the criteria of malignancy. Interpretation must be based on abundant and well-preserved cells. Knowledge of the entry point of the fine needle and a good clinical history can be paramount. Finally, the term "unsatisfactory" must be used judiciously, signifying a biopsy that cannot be evaluated.

THE REPORT

The ultimate aim of a cytologic report is the definitive diagnosis. This constitutes the correct and exact interpretation of the lesion and is couched in terms corresponding to those of histologic reports. Because a definitive diagnosis is not always possible, a meaningful descriptive diagnosis may be issued. For example, from a mass of the neck the findings of cells specific for lymphoid, salivary gland, or mesenchymal tissue may be important for clinical evaluation. Likewise, from a thickened area adjacent to a mastectomy site, a cell-sparse aspirate with no mammary parenchyma generally indicates scar tissue rather than recurrent tumor.

The clinician must understand the significance of the benign report. For example, periodic mammary NAB is especially appropriate for the patient with fibrocystic changes; from palpable breast lesions the false-negative rate is less than 2% in our institutions.

An unsatisfactory report, which no pathologist likes to generate, sometimes must be issued. This report informs the clinician that the specimen cannot be interpreted and, therefore, must be equated with NO BIOPSY. It is indicated for samples showing:

- Insufficient numbers of cells
- Numerous red blood or inflammatory cells that obscure underlying epithelial cells
- Cells distorted by drying or degeneration

CAVEAT

Biopsy by the fine needle frequently and correctly is equated with excisional biopsy. Decision-making and therapy can be based on aspiration biopsies. Yet, the sensitivity of the procedure in experienced hands and depending on the site and type of examination varies from approximately 80 to 96%. Therefore, appropriate care of the patient demands that with a suspicious clinical impression, a "benign" aspiration biopsy is no substitute for excisional biopsy.

PHILOSOPHY

At Lankenau Hospital, we have developed a philosophy based on our many years of experience with numerous and diverse specimens. Our philosophy stresses:

- Team approach
- Simplest equipment
- Papanicolaou technique
- Pattern evaluation with specific criteria

The team approach, synonymous with interaction among the pathologist, clinician, and radiologist, is essential for interpretation of the specimen. We believe that whenever possible, NAB should be performed by the clinician as a part of the initial examination of the lesion. Needle maneuvers frequently provide an extension of manual palpation, and the findings may alter decision-making for the patient. Unfortunately, without this approach the clinician sometimes first interprets as "benign" an "inconsequential" but actually malignant lesion, recommending "observation" rather than biopsy. Finally, this team approach provides essential checks and balances regarding patient care. The pathologist, however, must be cognizant of each aspect of the actual biopsy procedure and must be prepared to instruct the clinician at the bedside or in the laboratory by means of surgical or autopsy specimens. Prior to the final written report and as a vital segment of the team approach, we routinely discuss with the clinician each suspicious or positive interpretation, facilitating the application of the clinical data to the ABC.

The simplest equipment becomes mandatory when a heterogeneous group of clinicians performs the aspiration biopsy. Most of our 30,000 plus specimens have been procured with the 3-cc Luer-Lok syringe and 22-gauge needle. This ubiquitous, cost-effective tool presents no threat to the patient by virtue of its small size, in contrast to the patented syringe guns.

At Lankenau Hospital, all specimens are prepared according to the method of Papanicolaou. This is done principally because this procedure is familiar to both cytopathologists and cytotechnologists.

At the University of Alberta Hospitals, NAB had been sporadically performed on palpable lesions since 1972. It has gradually gained in popularity, and in the past 7 years the number of NABs has remained unchanged, with about 1000 aspirates from all sites yearly. As at Lankenau Hospital, the main staining technique used in our cytology laboratory is the Papanicolaou method. Staining with hematoxylin and eosin is performed when there is an excessive number of alcohol-fixed smears. Special stainings with mucicarmine, periodic acid-Schiff, or Fontana's method are used in selected cases. Air-dried smears are routinely stained by means of the May-Grünwald-Giemsa and/or Diff-Quick methods. In Europe, where aspiration biopsy has gained momentum, specimens frequently were taken by clinicians who were familiar with the air-dried, May-Grünwald-Giemsa technique. One procedure is not "better" than the other, and the choice must be left to individual preference as long as the final results are comparable.

The criteria of malignancy (see Diagnostic Criteria) have proved beneficial for the evaluation of our wide variety of specimens. The results are reproducible. They provide essential teaching tools for students, residents, cytotechnologists, and pathologists.

SUGGESTED READING

Berg JW, Robbins GF: A late look at the safety of aspiration biopsy. *Cancer* 1962;15:826–827.

Dahlgren SE, Nordenström B: *Transthoracic Needle Biopsy*. Chicago, Year Book Medical Publishers, 1966.

Kline TS: Aspiration biopsy of the lymph node: yea or nay? *Diagn Cytopathol* 1985;1:3–4.

Kline TS, Neal HS: Needle aspiration biopsy: a pilot study. JAMA 1978;239:36–39.

Kline TS: Communication and aspiration biopsy cytology: clear, concise, and to the point. *Diagn Cytopathol* 1990;6:153.

Kline TS: *Handbook of Fine Needle Aspiration Biopsy Cytology*, ed 2. New York, Churchill Livingstone, 1988.

Koss LG, Woyke S, Olszewski W: *Aspiration Biopsy: Cytologic Interpretation and Histologic Bases*. New York, Igaku-Shoin, 1984.

Lopes Cardozo P: *Atlas of Clinical Cytology*. Leyden, Targa's-Hertogenbosch, 1975.

Martin HE, Ellis EB: Biopsy by needle puncture and aspiration. *Ann Surg* 1930;92:169–181.

Roussel F, Dalion J, Benozio M: The risk of tumoral seeding in needle biopsies. *Acta Cytol* 1989;33:936–938.

Söderström N: *Fine-Needle Aspiration Biopsy*. New York, Grune & Stratton, 1966.

Stewart FW: The diagnosis of tumors by aspiration. *Am J Pathol* 1933;9:801–812.

2

CLINICAL AND LABORATORY PROCEDURES

In order to provide a good diagnostic cytology service, the interested hospital or private laboratory must have a well-organized cytology laboratory with competent personnel and a reasonable quality assurance program. A proper cytologic evaluation is only possible with an adequate and well-stained NAB sample.

To obtain an adequate cell sample all NABs must be performed by aspirators who are familiar with the technique. Usually, a superficial and palpable tumor is aspirated by a clinician during his or her physical examination. In some settings the biopsy is done by a cytopathologist in an Aspiration Biopsy Clinic. Nonpalpable lesions are almost always sampled by a radiologist under guidance of radiologic imaging.

BIOPSY PROCEDURE

Equipment

The basic tools for NAB consist of a needle and a syringe. The needle used is a disposable one with an outer diameter varying from 0.6 to 1.2 mm (23- to 18-gauge). The length of the needle varies from 3 to 20 cm, depending on the location of the lesion to undergo biopsy. For transthoracic and transabdominal NABs, a few types of long needle are commonly used:

—The Chiba needle is a sharply beveled, spinal-type 20- to 23-gauge needle.

—The Westcott needle has a slotted opening located at about 3 mm from the needle tip. The slot is used as a second cutting edge of the needle.

—The Rotex screw needle is a 19-gauge needle that has a stainless-steel screw needle measuring 0.55 mm located within the cannula. The needle screws into the lesion and samples its cells and tissue.

Regarding the syringe, many operators prefer a 3- or 5-ml plastic syringe for easy maneuverability. Others use 10- or 20-ml syringe for a stronger suction. Depending on the preference of the operator the NAB can be performed with or without a costly syringe holder or pistol that is commercially available.

Biopsy Technique

Palpable lesions. A superficially palpable mass lesion can be aspirated after sterilization of the skin by alcohol and fixation of the lesion between the thumb and index finger of one hand. The syringe with the needle is held with the other hand. Once the needle enters the lesion, negative pressure within the syringe is applied. To obtain an adequate cell sample the needle is moved up-and-down in at least three different directions with short stabs and/or a corkscrew motion (Fig. 2-1A). If the aspirate is seen in the hub of the needle, the negative pressure within the syringe is released to prevent diffusion of the biopsy material. The needle is then withdrawn from the lesion. It is disconnected from the syringe and then reconnected to permit

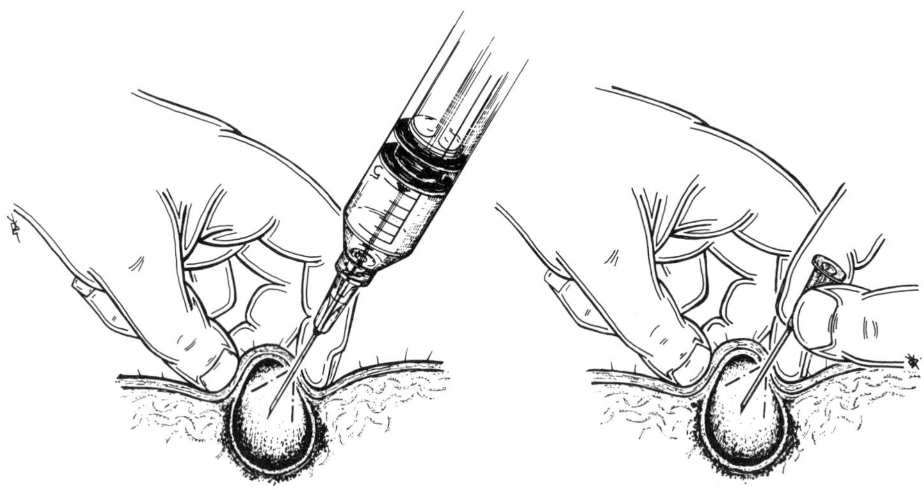

A B

Figure 2-1. A. Needle aspiration biopsy. **B.** Needle biopsy without aspiration.

entrance of an air column. Then by vigorous compression of the plunger, the specimen is expelled onto slides for preparation of direct smears. The needle and the syringe are washed with 2 milliliters of a balanced electrolyte solution that is subsequently used for preparation of cytocentrifuge smears or membrane filter preparations. The NAB generally should be repeated two or three times for procurement of adequate material. When a cystic lesion is aspirated, its liquid contents must be completely evacuated, and the lesion must be reexamined. If a residual tumor or mass is found, it should be aspirated, as a neoplasm may undergo extensive cystic degenerative changes, and examination of the cyst contents may reveal only necrotic debris and nondiagnostic cellular material. For a large tumor the NAB should be performed at the periphery of the neoplasm, as its central part usually undergoes necrosis.

Recently, a nonaspiration needle biopsy technique has been described to obtain cells from palpable mass lesions. The needle is inserted into the mass, and the cellular material is sucked into the needle by capillary permeability (Fig. 2-1B). A syringe is attached to discharge the sample onto the slide.

Other palpable lesions such as prostatic nodules and tumors of the female pelvis can be safely aspirated transrectally or transvaginally using a Franzen's instrument or a long spinal-type needle. The needle is molded to the finger and advanced into the lesion after digital palpation. The NAB then is performed as described for superficial lesions.

Nonpalpable lesions. NAB of these deeply located lesions requires special training and equipment. A detailed discussion on these procedures is beyond the scope of this concise book. Briefly, a biopsy is done on a mass lesion of the lung and mediastinum under the guidance of fluoroscopy with image intensification. If the biopsy is unsuccessful, ultrasonography (US) and computed tomography (CT) may be used to guide the needle. Space-occupying lesions of the pancreas, liver, kidneys, adrenals, and retroperitoneum are aspirated under US or CT guidance. Pelvic or retroperitoneal enlarged lymph nodes can accurately undergo biopsy under CT or fluoroscopic guidance. The latter method requires a nodal opacification by a pedal lymphangiography. A biopsy can be done on bone lesions under fluoroscopic or CT guidance. When the cortical bone appears intact a trocart fitted into a cannula is used to penetrate the surrounding soft tissue, periosteum, and cortex. When the lesion is reached, the pointed trocart is replaced by a trocart with a cutting edge, and both aspirate and core tissue are obtained. Superficially located, large lytic lesions can undergo biopsy without special equipment in the clinician's office. A deep-seated tumor of the brain can be accurately and safely biopsied using a stereotactic and CT-guided equipment.

COMPLICATIONS

Complications vary with the site undergoing biopsy, and they will be discussed in the following chapters. In general, all NABs may cause uncontrolled hemorrhage in patients with bleeding disorders. Seeding of cancer cells along the needle tract is generally a myth, with only a handful of cases reported. It is seen mainly in inoperable and diffuse tumors. Some specific complications are only encountered in transthoracic or transabdominal NABs.

Transthoracic NAB

Pneumothorax is the most common complication occurring in about 30% of patients who undergo this type of biopsy. Most cases of pneumothorax are asymptomatic and resolve spontaneously. However, about 5% of patients require a chest tube drainage. Transient hemotypsis occurs in about 5% of patients. Hemopericardium rarely happens in NAB of mediastinal lesions and requires pericardiocentesis. Other complications such as air embolism and vasovagal reactions are extremely rare. Needling of pulmonary arteries and veins, aorta, and even an aortic aneurysm does not cause any serious bleeding.

Transabdominal NAB

This biopsy technique is safe and is rarely associated with major complications. Although a number of hollow organs and large blood vessels are perforated during the procedure, peritonitis and intraabdominal bleeding are exceedingly rare complications. Acute pancreatitis and intrahepatic hematoma requiring surgical evacuation are extremely rare.

PREPARATION OF SPECIMENS

Direct Smear

A drop of aspirated material is deposited near the frosted end of a glass slide and is gently smeared using a cover slip or another glass slide. If the material is markedly diluted with blood, cellular elements should be concentrated by means of one of the techniques outlined by Kline, Abele et al., or Hidvegi. The prepared smears are immediately fixed in 95% ethanol or by a commercial spray fixative for staining by the Papanicolaou technique, with hematoxylin and eosin or by other special and immunocytochemical staining procedures. They may also be air-dried for staining with one of the modified Romanowsky staining methods, such as the May-Grünwald-Giemsa or Diff-Quik techniques.

Cytocentrifuge Smear

The cell suspension is obtained by washing the biopsy needle and syringe with 2 ml of a balanced electrolyte solution. Depending on the cell concentration two to ten drops of the solution are put in each chamber of a Cytospin II (Shandon Instruments) and centrifuged at 1500 rpm for 5 minutes. If the button is too thick, it should be smeared with a coverslip or slide, and the prepared smears should then be rapidly fixed in 95% ethanol prior to staining with one of different methods as described above. Cytocentrifuge smears are convenient for special stains.

Membrane Filtrate

The saline suspension is slowly funneled through a Millipore filter (19 × 42 mm, pore size 5-μm, Millipore Corp.) premoistened with 95% ethanol. This is accomplished by a vacuum-attached system. Before the vacuum is stopped, a few drops of 95% ethanol are added. The filter is then removed and fixed in ethanol from 2 minutes to overnight. Thereafter, it is stained by the Papanicolaou method, with the exception of final clearing in absolute isopropyl alcohol rather than ethanol.

Cell Block

When all necessary smears have been prepared, the remaining material in the centrifuge tube is used for cell block preparation. Agar may be used to entrap cells and tissue fragments that will be processed according to the routine histologic techniques. Tissue sections from the cell block are better for the demonstration of intracytoplasmic antigens by immunocytochemical methods.

Electron Microscopic Study

Tissue fragments aspirated are the best materials for electron microscopic study. They should be removed rapidly from the aspirate and fixed in 2 or 4% glutaraldehyde. They are then postfixed in osmium tetroxide for 30 minutes and embedded in epoxy-araldite. Suspended cells are simply pelleted out of the balanced salt solution and prepared according to the technique developed by Akhtar et al. for ultrastructural studies.

ROUTINE STAINING METHODS

Different staining methods have their advantages and disadvantages. The Papanicolaou preparation and staining with hematoxylin and eosin are excellent for assessment of nuclear chromatin and visualization of cytoplasmic keratin. The May-Grünwald-Giemsa and Diff-Quik techniques are good for typing lymphohematopoietic cells and for demonstration of secretory products in the epithelial cell cytoplasm and the matrix on the smear background. Usually, the evaluation of both fixed and air-dried cellular materials is helpful in making an accurate cytodiagnosis.

Ethanol-fixed smears are routinely stained by means of the Papanicolaou method or with hematoxylin and eosin. Special staining with periodic acid-Schiff, mucicarmine, Prussian blue, or by means of the Fontana and Grimelius methods is also performed on wet-fixed smears for the demonstration of particular intracytoplasmic materials; generally destaining is unnecessary. Air-dried smears can be stained with oil red-O for the detection of intracytoplasmic fat.

IMMUNOCYTOCHEMICAL STAINING METHODS

Ethanol-fixed smears are suitable for most studies, although specially prepared specimens must be obtained for hormone-receptor demonstration. The majority of these studies may also be performed on ethanol-fixed slides. Peroxidase-antiperoxidase and avidin-biotin are two techniques used in cytology. A number of antisera to different types of intracytoplasmic intermediate filament protein may be used to further type aspirated tumor cells. It should be borne in mind that immunocytochemical staining is compounded with diagnostic pitfalls and, therefore, both known positive and negative controls should be run simultaneously with the im-

Table 2-1. Commonly Used Antisera in Tumor Typing

ANTISERUM	TUMOR
Epithelial membrane antigen	Epithelial tumors
Carcinoembryonic antigen	Epithelial tumors
Leukocyte common antigen and leukocyte subsets	Lymphoma
S-100 protein	Melanoma, neural tumors, lipomatous tumors
Neuron-specific enolase	Neuroendocrine tumors
Peptide hormones (e.g., insulin, glucagon, etc.)	Endocrine tumors of the pancreas
Calcitonin	Medullary carcinoma of the thyroid
Thyroglobulin	Thyroid epithelial tumors
Alpha-fetoprotein	York sac tumor, embryonal carcinoma, hepatocellular carcinoma
β-human chorionic gonadotropin	Germ cell tumors
Prostatic acid phosphatase and prostate-specific antigen	Prostatic carcinomas
Lysozyme	Histiocytic tumors
Factor VIII-related antigen	Endothelial cell tumors
Myoglobin	Striated muscle tumors
Intermediate filaments	
Keratin	Epithelial tumors, mesothelioma
Vimentin	Mesenchymal tumors, some epithelial tumors
Desmin	Muscle tumors
Glial fibrillary acid protein	Gliomas
Neurofilaments	Neural tumors

munocytochemical tests chosen to study the case. As a rule, immunostaining using a battery of antisera should be ordered in all cases studied. Some commonly used antisera and their diagnostic value in ABC are listed in Table 2-1.

SUGGESTED READING

Abele JS, Miller TR, King EB, et al.: Smearing techniques for the concentration of particles from fine needle aspiration biopsy. *Diagn Cytopathol* 1985;1:59–65

Akhtar M, Ali MA, Huq M, et al.: Fine needle biopsy: comparison of cellular yield with and without aspiration. *Diagn Cytopathol* 1989;5:162–165.

Akhtar M, Barkry M, Nash EJ: An improved method for processing fine needle aspiration biopsy for electron microscopy. *Am J Clin Pathol* 1986;85:57–60.

Hidvegi FD: *Guides to Clinical Aspiration Biopsy. Liver and Pancreas.* New York, Igaku-Shoin, pp 17–26.

Kline TS: *Handbook of Fine Needle Aspiration Biopsy Cytology*, ed 2. New York, Churchill Livingstone, 1988, pp 9–16.

Nguyen GK: What is the value of fine needle aspiration biopsy in the cytodiagnosis of soft tissue tumors? *Diagn Cytopathol* 1988;4:352–355

Tao LC: *Guides to Clinical Aspiration Biopsy. Lung, Pleura and Mediastinum.* New York, Igaku-Shoin, 1988, pp 11–17.

Ramaekers FCS, Vooijs GP, Huijsmans ACLM, et al.: Immunohistochemistry as an aid in diagnostic cytopathology. In DeLellis RA *Advances in Immunohistochemistry.* New York, Raven Press, 1988, pp 133–163.

Zajdela A, Zillhardt P, Voillemot N: Cytologic diagnosis by fine needle sampling without aspiration. *Cancer* 1987;59:1201–1205.

3

BREAST

A palpable breast lesion is a common finding in women. It may be caused by a tumor or an inflammatory process. Aspiration biopsy for cytologic evaluation of breast lumps is a rapid, inexpensive, and accurate method of clinical investigation. In many places with considerable experience, a mastectomy has been performed on the basis of positive ABC, obviating an intraoperative frozen section diagnosis. However, the cytodiagnosis of breast cancers has diagnostic pitfalls and requires experience.

INDICATIONS AND CONTRAINDICATIONS FOR NAB

NAB of breast lumps has virtually no contraindication. The technique may be used to confirm a recurrent or inoperable breast cancer prior to radiotherapy, chemotherapy, or hormonal manipulation. It is also useful in diagnosing a breast lump of unknown nature. Nonpalpable breast lesions detected by mammography may be successfully aspirated under guidance of stereotactic equipment and diagnosed cytologically.

BENIGN NONNEOPLASTIC LESIONS

Inflammatory Disorders

Acute mastitis is a bacterial infection spreading in the ductal system of the mammary gland. It is commonly seen during the breast feeding period, and its

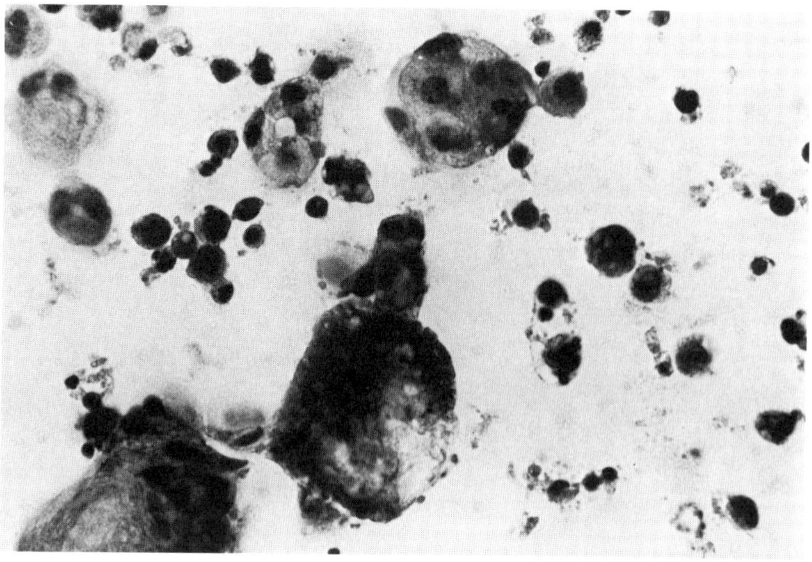

Figure 3-1. Fat necrosis showing numerous lipophages and inflammatory cells. (Papanicolaou ×250.)

diagnosis usually does not require morphologic confirmation. NAB of the breast reveals necrotic debris and inflammatory exudate.

Plasma cell mastitis is rarely encountered in clinical practice. It may mimic a breast cancer on physical examination. NAB of the lesion in the early phase of the disease shows numerous plasma cells, polymorphonuclear leukocytes, lymphoid cells, and macrophages, as well as groups of atypical acinar cells and fragments of ductal epithelium with mild atypias. During the healing phase the lesion becomes fibrotic and yields in NAB only a few plasma cells and lymphoid cells.

Fat necrosis of the breast usually follows a blunt trauma or surgery to the gland. It may simulate a breast cancer clinically. NAB reveals necrotic fatty tissue, inflammatory cells, and lipophages with vacuolated cytoplasm (Fig. 3-1). Growing fibroblasts with bizarre nuclei may also be seen.

Fibrocystic Changes

Fibrocystic changes of the breast are common in adult women and encompass a wide variety of morphologic features characterized by a mixture of cystic formation and fibrosis, ductal and lobular epithelial hyperplasia, and sclerosing adenosis. Each of these three components may be predominant. Cysts and fibrosis are the most frequent lesions. In large cysts, the epithelial lining may be flattened or atrophic. Not uncommonly, it undergoes apocrine metaplastic changes with epithelial proliferation and papillary projections. NAB of a large cyst with atrophic epithelium reveals turbid liquid containing necrotic debris. An apocrine cyst yields, in addition, fragments of apocrine metaplastic epithelium with granular, eosinophilic,

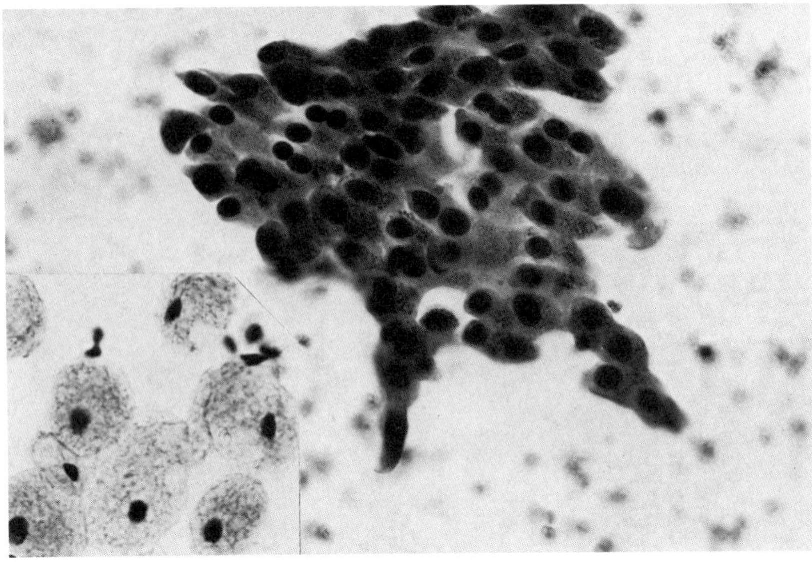

Figure 3-2. Fibrocystic changes showing a sheet of apocrine metaplastic epithelium. Note granular well-defined cytoplasm. **Inset:** benign foam cells. (Papanicolaou ×250)

abundant, well-defined cytoplasm, and vesicular nuclei showing conspicuous nucleoli (Fig. 3-2). Occasionally, these cells display remarkable nuclear atypias mimicking those of an apocrine carcinoma (Fig. 3-3).

Ductal epithelial hyperplasia is characterized by irregular folding sheets of

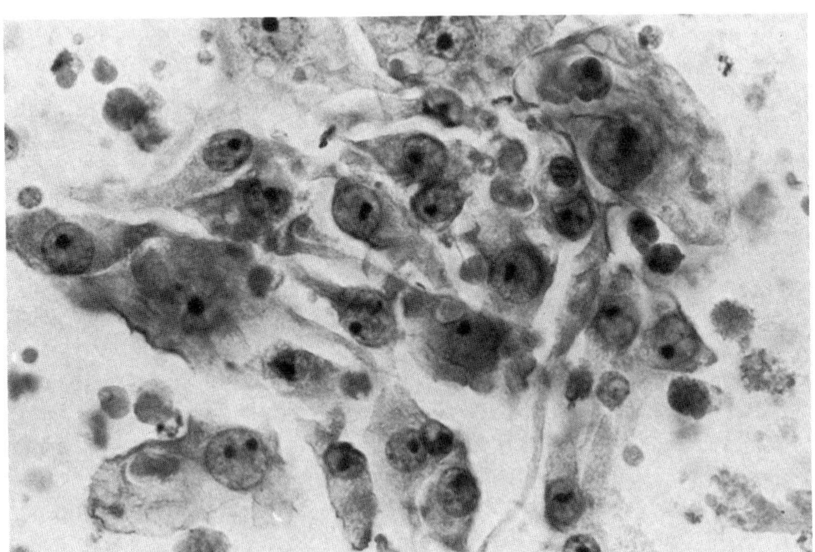

Figure 3-3. A cluster of atypical apocrine metaplastic cells. Note the well-defined cytoplasm and macronucleoli. (Papanicolaou ×400.)

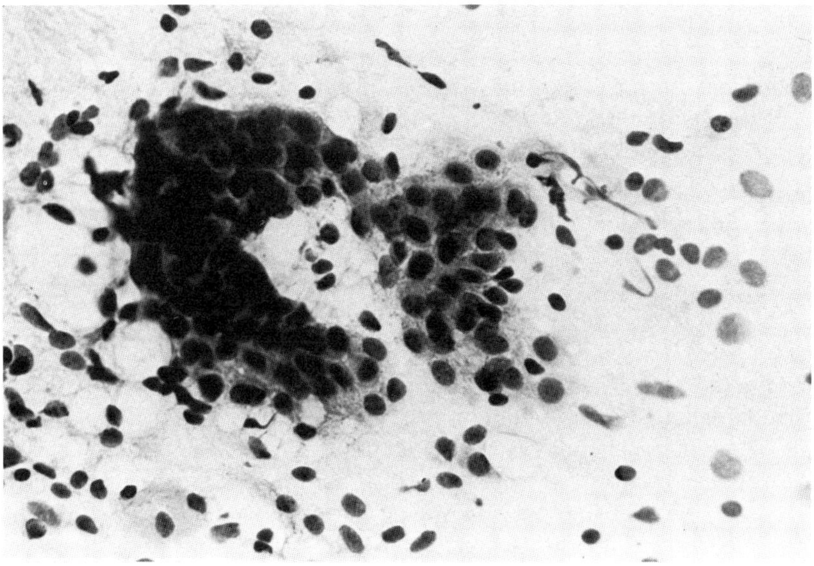

Figure 3-4. Ductal epithelial hyperplasia. An irregular fragment of slightly hyperplastic benign ductal epithelium and numerous scattered naked nuclei of myoepithelial cells. (Papanicolaou ×250.)

glandular epithelium with a honeycomb pattern (Fig. 3-4). Irregular monolayered epithelial sheets are seen in ABC of a sclerosing adenosis (Fig. 3-5). In the two later situations, epithelial fragments contain identifiable myoepithelial cells. The smear background displays numerous bipolar naked nuclei of myoepithelial cells.

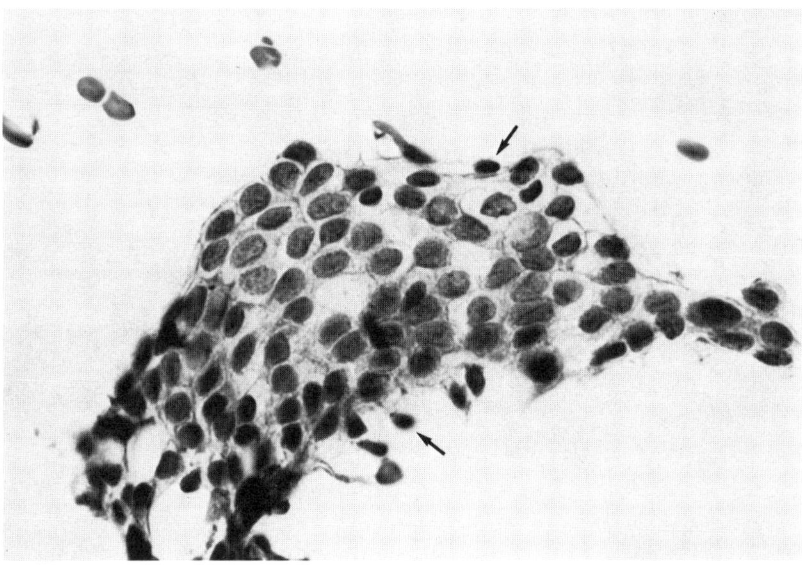

Figure 3-5. A fragment of benign ductal epithelium containing myoepithelial cells (*arrow*) aspirated from a sclerosing adenosis. (Papanicolaou ×400.)

BENIGN TUMORS

Fibroadenoma is the commonest benign breast tumor occurring chiefly in young women. In the majority of cases fibroadenoma can be diagnosed clinically and does not need morphologic confirmation by ABC. NAB of a classic fibroadenoma yields highly cellular material consisting of several irregularly branching epithelial fragments with tightly packed cells (fronds) and cells in a honeycomb pattern. Numerous hyperchromatic, bipolar, and naked nuclei of myoepithelial cells are dispersed throughout the slide (Fig. 3-6). Epithelial cells may show marked nuclear atypias, and mesenchymal cells are rarely seen in the aspirate.

Cystosarcoma phylloides, or giant fibroadenoma of the breast, may be classified as benign or malignant, depending on the morphologic features of the tumor stromal cells. The term malignant cystosarcoma phylloides is reserved for such a tumor having a fibrosarcomatous stroma. ABC of a benign cystosarcoma phylloides is similar to that of a fibroadenoma. However, abundant stromal elements are seen (Fig. 3-7). The cytodiagnosis of a malignant cystosarcoma phylloides may be suggested when the aspirated stromal cells show features of malignant fibroblasts (Fig. 3-8).

Intraductal papilloma rarely manifests as a breast lump. In almost all cases the neoplasm is associated with a bloody nipple discharge that shows clusters of benign epithelial cells. NAB from a palpable ductal papilloma reveals large and tight groups or sheets of columnar or cuboidal epithelial cells showing well-defined cytoplasm and round or vesicular nuclei with conspicuous nucleoli. Myoepithelial cells are

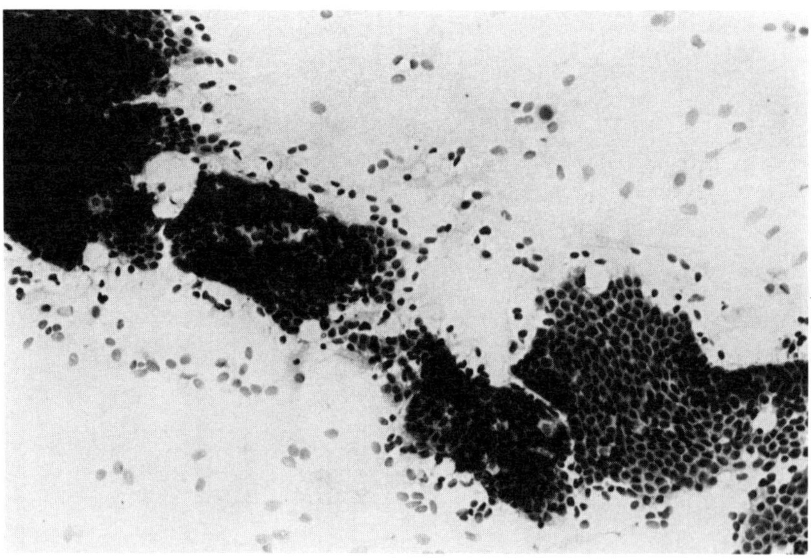

Figure 3-6. Fibroadenoma showing irregularly branching epithelial fragments with tightly packed cells. Note the honeycomb pattern and several naked nuclei of myoepithelial cells. (Papanicolaou ×100.)

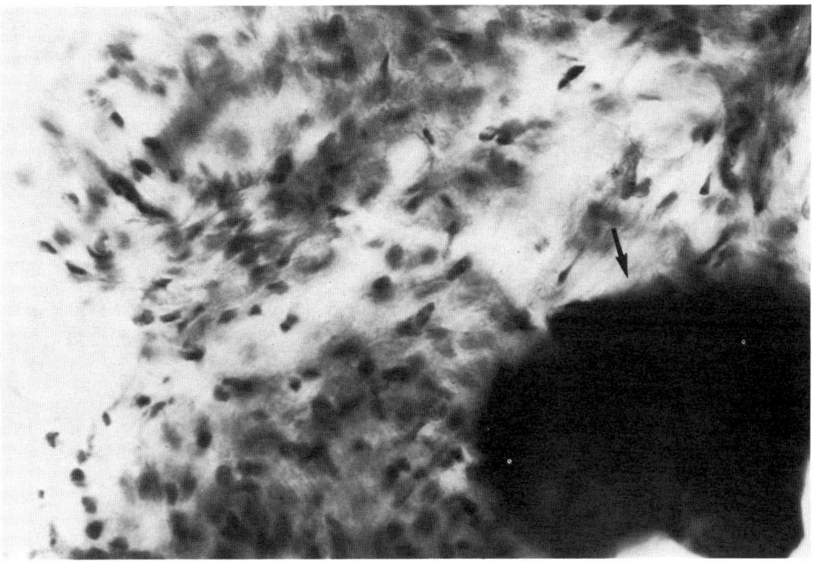

Figure 3-7. Benign cytosarcoma phylloides. Note fragments of edematous stromal tissue containing numerous fibroblasts and a thick fragment of ductal epithelium (*arrow*). (Papanicolaou ×250.)

seen in the tumor epithelial fragments and on the smear background. (Fig. 3-9). The cytologic differential diagnosis between an intraductal papilloma (especially the so-called subareolar papillomatosis) and a papillary carcinoma of the breast can be very difficult, and the final diagnosis should be made on histologic examination of the excised tumor.

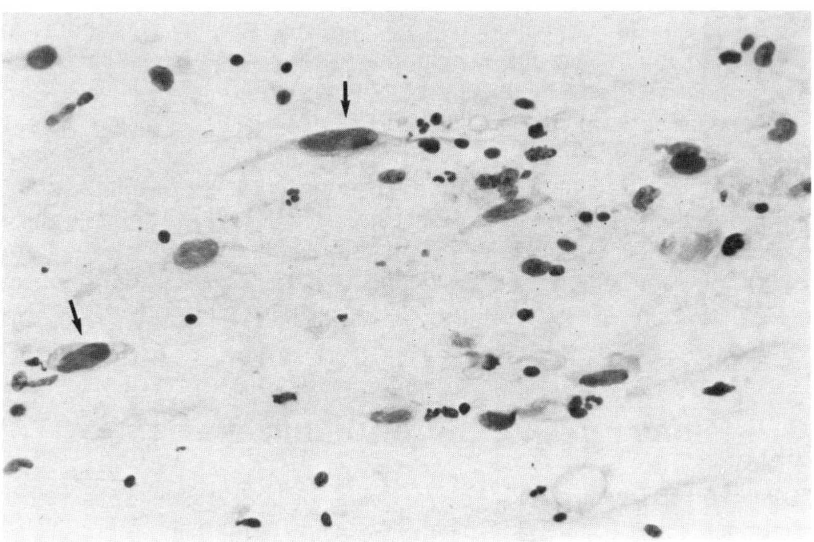

Figure 3-8. Malignant cytosarcoma phylloides. Note pleomorphic spindle-shaped fibroblasts (*arrow*). (Papanicolaou ×300.)

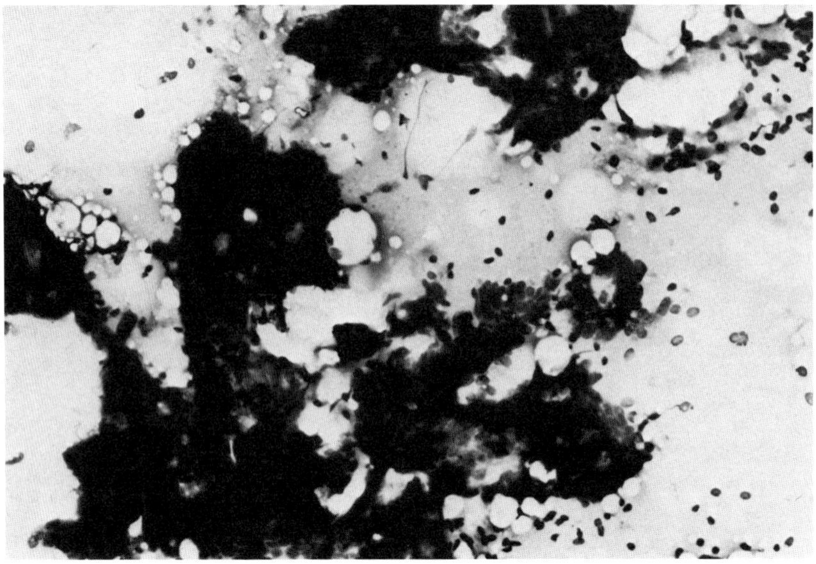

Figure 3-9. Intraductal papilloma. Note thick papillary fragments of benign columnar epithelium showing strong cellular cohesiveness. Numerous naked nuclei of myoepithelial cells are also seen. (Diff-Quik ×100.)

MALIGNANT TUMORS

Ductal Carcinoma

Ductal carcinomas constitute about 80% of all breast cancers and have several variants, such as medullary, mucinous, apocrine, and papillary carcinomas. In general, ABC of an infiltrating duct carcinoma of the breast is cellular and shows numerous single and loosely clustered malignant glandular cells with macronucleoli. The smear background usually shows necrotic debris. Thick tridimensional clusters of tumor cells are present, but they are almost always accompanied by dispersed cancer cells at the periphery. The tumor cells show a variable amount of cytoplasm, and their nuclei are round or vesicular and display a variable chromasia and macronucleoli (Fig. 3-10). Cells showing more abundant cytoplasm, intracytoplasmic vacuoles containing condensed mucous globules, and cells arranged in an Indian-file pattern may be seen on rare occasions (Fig. 3-11).

Common Ductal Carcinoma Variants

Medullary carcinoma usually yields sheets of large cancer cells with fragile cytoplasm and nuclei containing macronucleoli. Additionally, there are varying numbers of bizarre naked nuclei. Numerous lymphoid cells are present (Fig. 3-12).

Mucinous carcinoma is characterized by tight clusters or balls of cancer cells in a mucinous background. Psammoma bodies are occasionally observed (Fig. 3-13).

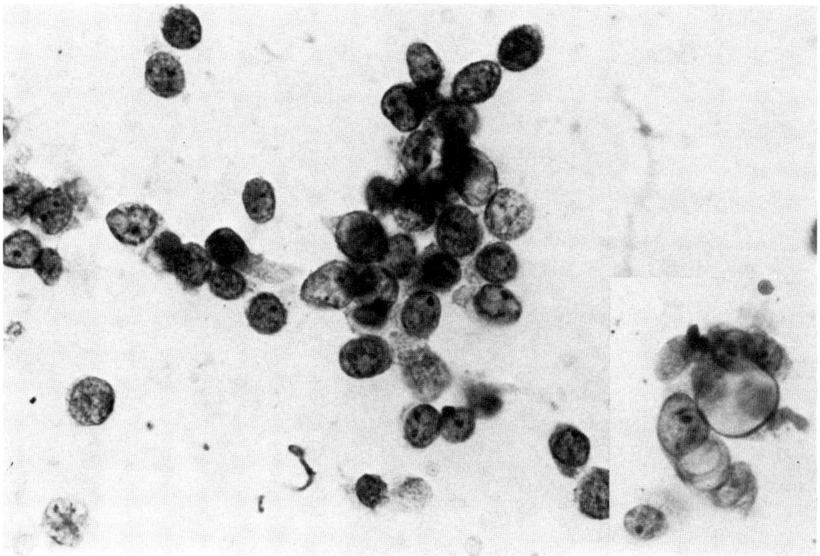

Figure 3-10. Infiltrating duct carcinoma showing dyshesive and irregular clusters of tumor cells. **Inset:** tumor cells with vacuolated cytoplasm. (Papanicolaou ×400.)

The specimen is cell-rich and also contains dyshesive sheets and clusters of tumor cells. Nuclear changes are inconspicuous.

Apocrine cell carcinoma shows abundant large cells singly and in loose syncytial clusters. The cells show a granular, ill-defined cytoplasm and vesicular nuclei with macronucleoli. Necrotic debris is often seen (Fig. 3-14).

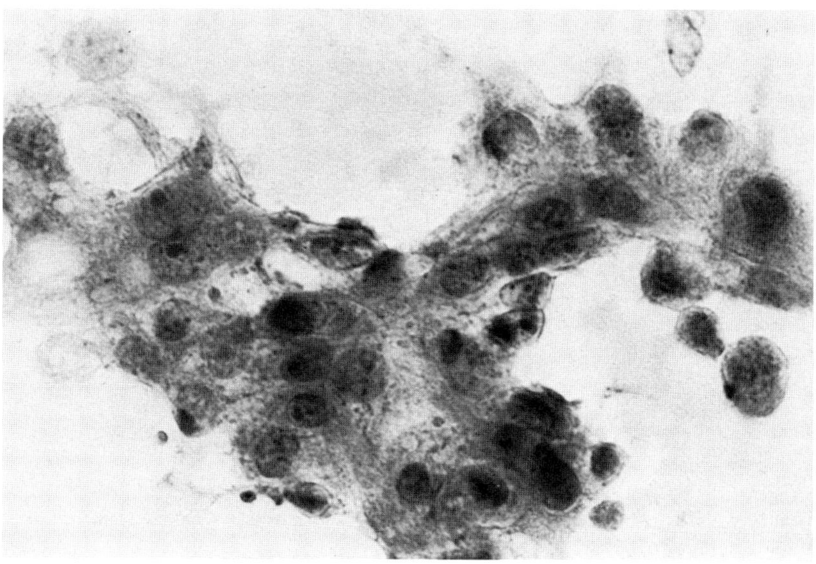

Figure 3-11. Infiltrating duct carcinoma showing a cluster of tumor cells displaying variable, ill-defined cytoplasm and slightly pleomorphic nuclei with macronucleoli. (Papanicolaou ×400.)

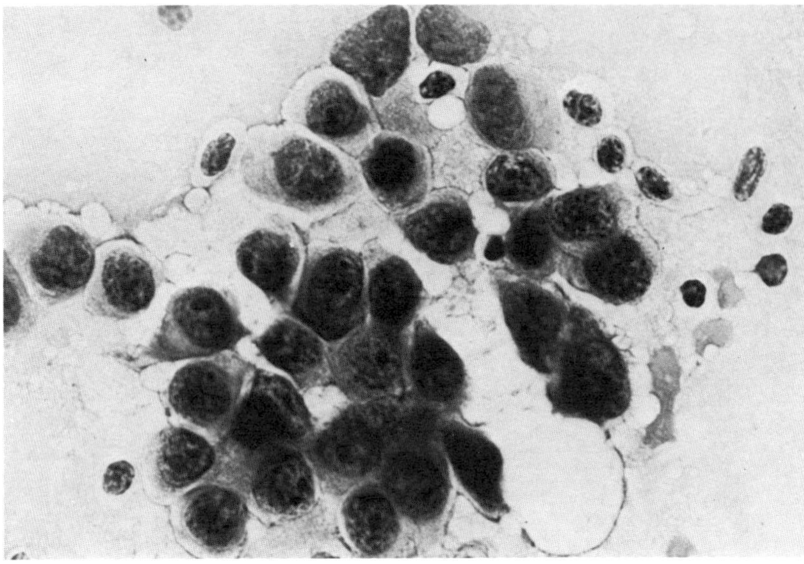

Figure 3-12. Medullary carcinoma showing lymphocytes and large dyshesive cancer cells containing macronucleoli. (Papanicolaou ×400.)

Papillary carcinoma usually yields numerous cancer cells in sheets or papillary clusters. The tumor cells are monomorphic, columnar, or cuboidal and show round or vesicular nuclei with inconspicuous nucleoli. Hemosiderin-laden macrophages are usually present. However, myoepithelial cells are absent (Fig. 3-15).

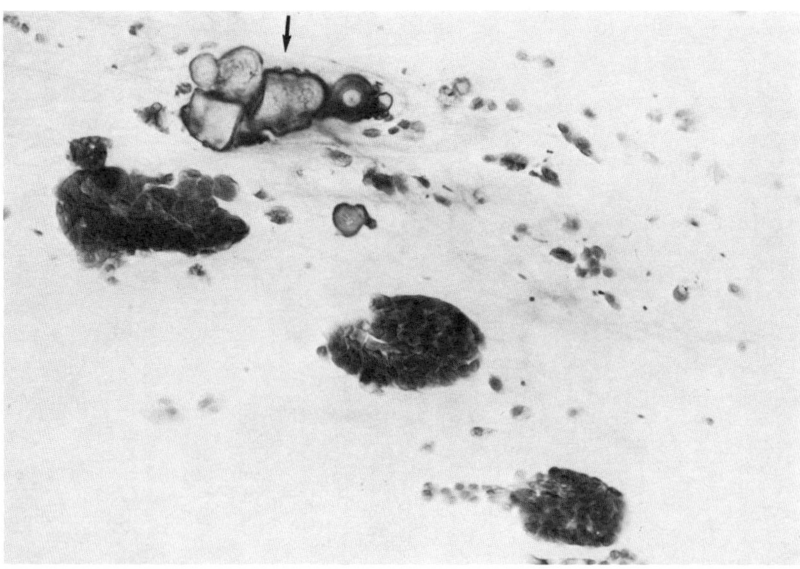

Figure 3-13. Mucinous carcinoma showing tight "balls" of cancer cells in a mucoid background. Psammoma bodies are present (*arrow*). (Papanicolaou ×100.)

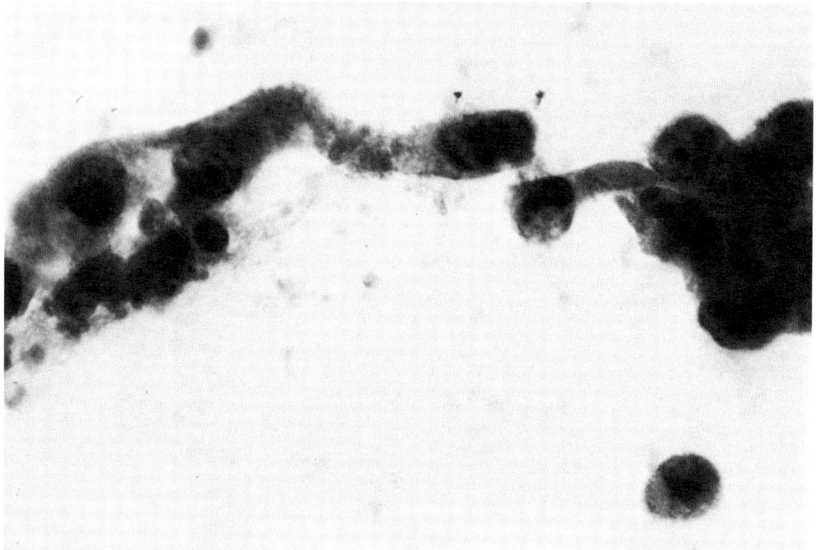

Figure 3-14. Apocrine cell carcinoma. Note single and loose groups of tumor cells showing ill-defined, abundant granular cytoplasm and macronucleoli. (Papanicolaou ×400.)

Lobular Carcinoma

Infiltrating lobular carcinomas constitute approximately 20% of all breast cancers. They usually show in NAB scanty cellular material. The tumor cells are seen singly, in loose clusters, and in short chains (Indian files) (Fig. 3-16). They are

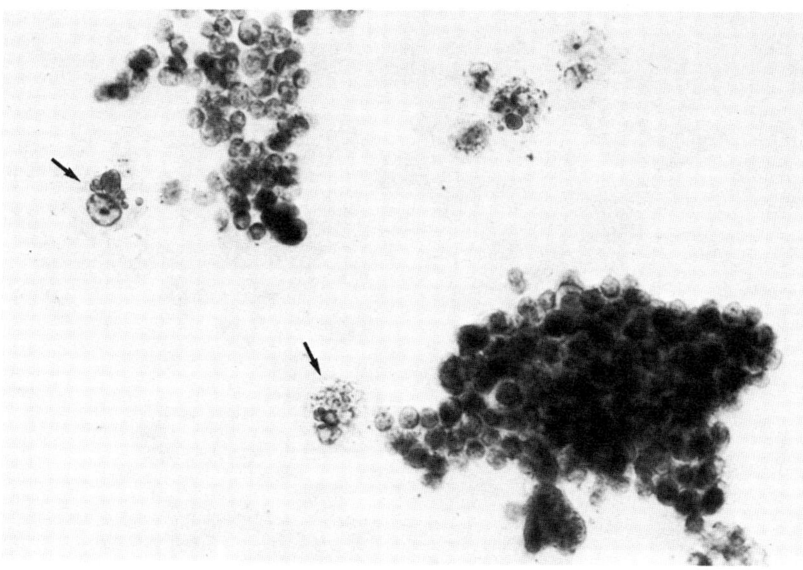

Figure 3-15. Papillary carcinoma. Note tumor cells in tight clusters. Hemosiderin-laden macrophages are seen (*arrow*). (Papanicolaou ×250.)

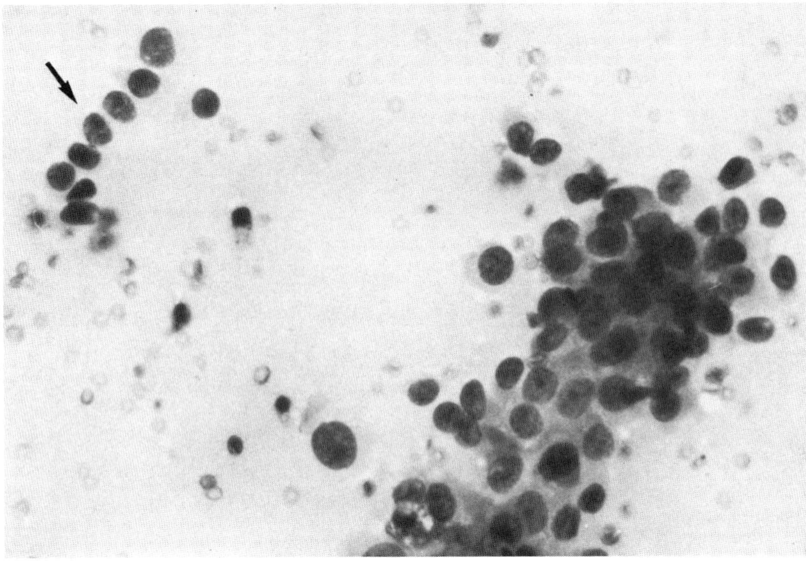

Figure 3-16. Lobular carcinoma showing regular tumor cells singly, in dyshesive clusters, and in Indian-file arrangement (*arrow*). (Papanicolaou ×400.)

polygonal in shape with little cytoplasm and eccentrically located nuclei showing a finely granular chromatin pattern and fairly conspicuous nucleoli. Tumor cells displaying intracytoplasmic vacuoles with condensed mucous globules are more commonly seen than in ABC of ductal carcinoma cases (Fig. 3-17).

Cytologic features of some common breast carcinomas are summarized in Table 3-1.

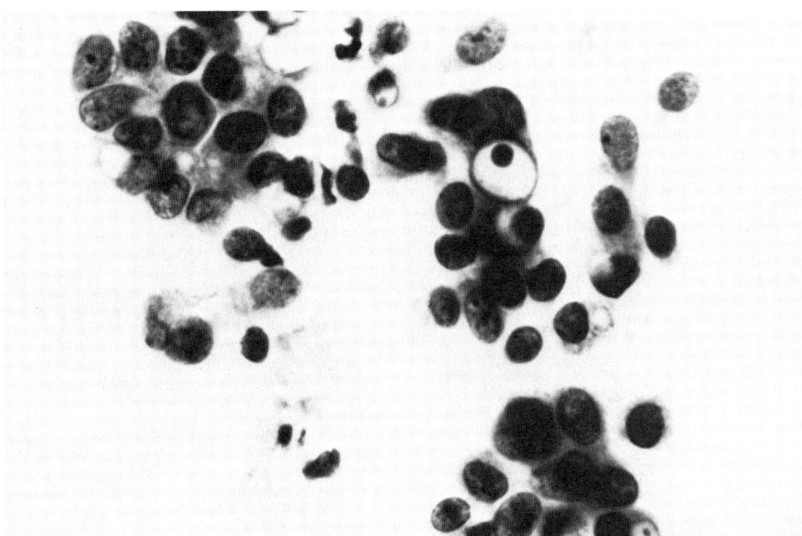

Figure 3-17. Lobular carcinoma. Note tumor cells with intracytoplasmic vacuoles containing condensed mucous globules. (Hemotoxylin and eosin ×400.)

Table 3-1. Cytomorphology of Common Breast Carcinomas

ABC	DUCTAL CARCINOMA (NOS)	MEDULLARY CARCINOMA	MUCINOUS CARCINOMA	PAPILLARY CARCINOMA	LOBULAR CARCINOMA
Cell arrangement	Dyshesive clusters of moderate-sized cells	Syncytia, large cells	Cell balls	Papillary aggregates	Isolated small cells
Tumor cells					
Anisonucleosis	+++	+++	+	+	+
Irregular nuclei	+++	+++	+	+	+
Macronucleoli	++	+++	+	+	+
Other features		Pleomorphic cells Naked nuclei Lymphocytes	Mucinous material	Hemosiderin-laden macrophages	Indian filling Cytoplasmic mucous globules

Other Breast Cancers

All types of malignant nonepithelial tumor may occur in the mammary glands. Of these, malignant cystosarcoma phylloides is the commonest, while angiosarcoma is the rarest. NAB from an angiosarcoma of the breast reveals numerous blood cells and tight and loose clusters of pleomorphic and spindle-shaped cancer cells that may stain positively with factor VIII-related antigen antiserum. Metastatic carcinomas to the breast are also unusual, with carcinomas of the ovary, lung, and kidney and cutaneous malignant melanoma the most common primaries.

DIAGNOSTIC ACCURACY AND PITFALLS

In experienced hands ABC of palpable breast lesions may have a diagnostic accuracy reaching 95%. However, both false-negative and false-positive diagnoses may occur.

A false-negative diagnostic rate for breast cancers of up to 20% has been reported. The main reasons are inadequate sampling (faulty biopsy technique) and lack of experience in dealing with aspirates containing scanty malignant cells.

False-positive diagnoses have severe consequences and are usually the results of misinterpretation of benign cells as malignant cells because of the lack of experience.

SUGGESTED READING

Consensus Statement by the Cancer Committee of the College of American Pathologists: is "fibrocystic disease" of the breast precancerous? *Arch Pathol Lab Med* 1986;100:171–173.

Eisenberg AJ, Hajdu SI, Wilhelms J, et al.: Preoperative aspiration cytology of breast tumors. *Acta Cytol* 1986;30:135–146.

Frable WJ: Needle aspiration of the breast. *Cancer* 1984;53:671-676.

Grant CS, Goellner JR, Welch JS, et al.: Fine needle aspiration of the breast. *Mayo Clin Proc* 1986;61:377–381.

Kline TS: Masquerades of malignancy. A review of 4241 aspirates from the breast. *Acta Cytol* 1981;25:263–266.

Kline TS, Kannan V, Kline IK: Appraisal and cytomorphologic analysis of common carcinomas of the breast. *Diagn Cytopathol* 1985;1:188–193.

Kline TS, Kannan V: Papillary carcinoma of the breast: a cytomorphologic analysis. *Arch Pathol Lab Med* 1986;110:189–191.

Kline TS, Kline IK: *Guides to Clinical Aspiration Biopsy. Breast.* New York, Igaku-Shoin, 1989.

Koss LG, Woyke S, Olszewski W: The breast. In *Aspiration Biopsy. Cytologic Interpretation and Histologic Bases.* New York, Igaku-Shoin, 1984, pp 53–104.

Rosenthal DL: Breast lesions diagnosed by fine needle aspiration. *Pathol Res Pract* 1986;181:645–656.

4

THYROID AND PARATHYROID

THYROID

NAB of the thyroid for cytologic evaluation of thyroid lesions is a routine diagnostic procedure. It proves to be useful in confirming the clinical diagnosis of a thyroid disease. It can diminish the myriad of costly laboratory tests. Finally, it is the most cost-effective and available method for identifying thyroid tumors.

Indications and Contraindications for NAB

The main indication for NAB of the thyroid is the presence of a nodule that is suspected of being a neoplasm. The technique is also used to confirm a benign cyst of the gland or a suspected thyroiditis. The thyroid NAB is contraindicated in patients with bleeding disorders.

Normal Thyroid

About 10% of all palpable thyroid nodules have no structural abnormality. NAB of an otherwise normal thyroid tissue reveals numerous follicular epithelial cells present in groups of variable size or in monolayered sheets showing a honeycomb pattern. Rarely, a whole thyroid follicle may be seen. The individual cells have a finely granular and ill-defined cytoplasm and round or oval nuclei with a finely granular chromatin pattern. Colloid material is present in small amounts as isolated

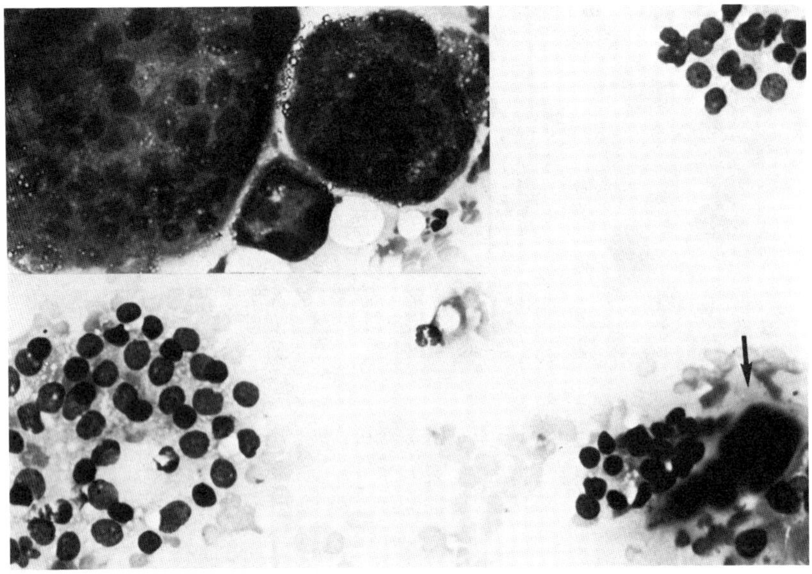

Figure 4-1. Normal thyroid ABC showing irregular fragment of colloid material (*arrow*), fragments of follicular epithelium with honeycomb pattern. **Inset:** intact thyroid follicles. (MGG ×250.)

irregular fragments or strands of granular material that stain blue with the May-Grünwald-Giemsa (MGG) technique. With the Papanicolaou method it variably stains orange, green, or yellow. The background of the smear is rich in blood cells (Fig. 4-1).

Thyroid Cysts

Thyroglossal duct cyst is the commonest congenital anomaly, and it is located on the midline of the neck. NAB from a noninfected cyst usually reveals a small amount of yellow fluid containing single and clustered benign squamous cells and a few inflammatory cells.

Noncongenital cystic lesions of the thyroid result from hemorrhagic necrosis of a colloid nodule or a thyroid tumor. Thus, cytologic examination of the cystic content is mandatory. NAB of a long-standing, benign thyroid cyst usually shows a variable amount of colloid material, benign foam cells, and hemosiderin-laden macrophages (Fig. 4-2).

Thyroiditis

Acute pyogenic thyroiditis is rarely seen in clinical practice. Its diagnosis is usually made by means of physical examination. NAB from the inflamed gland reveals necrotic debris and numerous polymorphonuclear leukocytes.

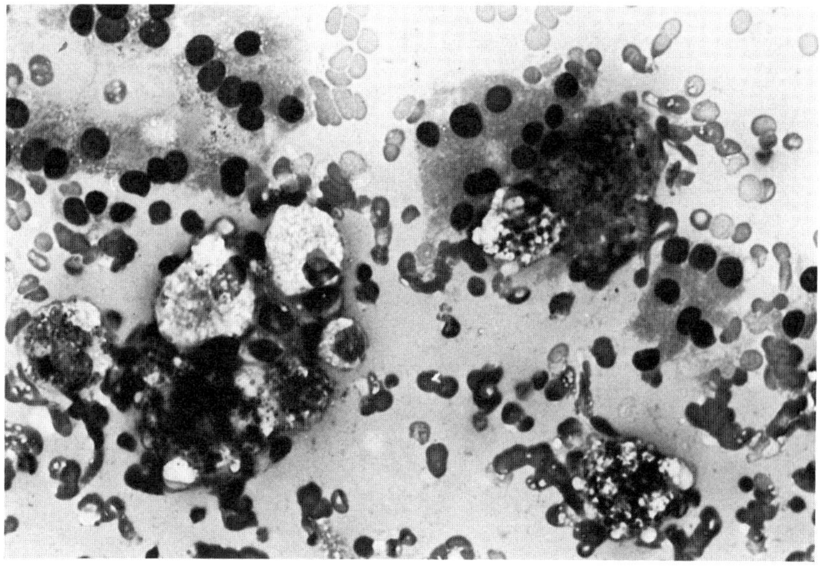

Figure 4-2. Benign thyroid cyst showing numerous foam cells. (MGG ×250.)

Subacute thyroiditis, or de Quervain's thyroiditis, is uncommon and occurs mainly in adult women. The gland is enlarged and painful. It yields in needle aspirates clusters of epithelioid cells with ill-defined cytoplasm and carrot-shaped or elongated nuclei, large multinucleated giant cells, and mature lymphoid cells (Fig. 4-3). Degenerated follicular epithelial cells may be seen.

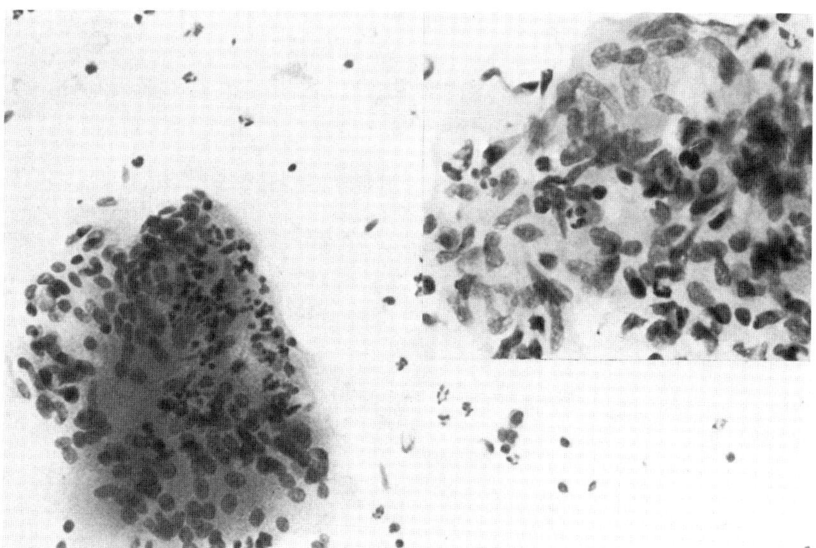

Figure 4-3. Subacute thyroiditis. A large multinucleated giant cell. **Inset:** A large cluster of epithelioid cells. (Papanicolaou ×100, **Inset** ×250.)

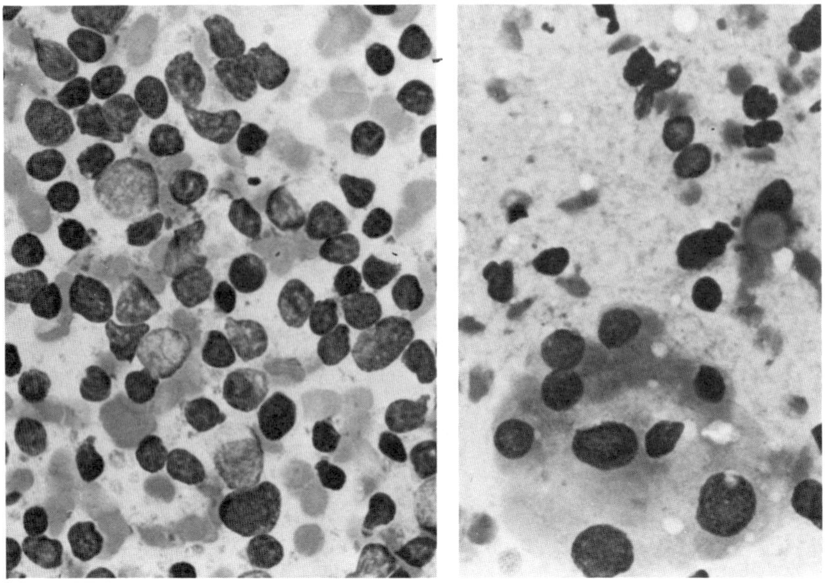

A B

Figure 4-4. Hashimoto's disease. **A.** Lymphoid cells at different stages of maturation. **B.** A cluster of Hürthle cells. (MGG ×400.)

Chronic lymphocytic thyroiditis, or Hashimoto's disease, is a common thyroid disorder in middle-aged women. The gland is often symmetrically enlarged, rubbery, and painless. NAB of the gland reveals numerous lymphoid cells at different stages of maturation, clusters of follicular epithelial cells, and a variable number of Hürthle cells, which are actually transformed follicular cells. They show abundant granular and eosinophilic cytoplasm. On rare occasions, the Hürthle cells are pleomorphic and display bizarre nuclei with prominent nucleoli mimicking cancer cells (Fig 4-4A and B). In advanced stages, the thyroid is fibrotic and yields only a small number of lymphoid cells and a few fibroblasts.

Riedel's struma, or invasive fibrotic thyroiditis, is a very rare condition. The affected thyroid is wooden hard and in NAB usually yields acellular material or a few fibroblasts.

Cellular features of different types of thyroiditis are summarized in Table 4-1.

Hyperplasia

Hyperplasia of follicular epithelial cells of the thyroid occurs principally in two conditions: Graves' disease and colloid nodular goiter.

Graves' disease, or toxic diffuse goiter, is a primary hyperthyroidism affecting mainly middle-aged women. The thyroid is usually diffusely enlarged but, rarely, a palpable nodule may be present. NAB of the gland reveals little or no colloid material and groups of hyperplastic follicular cells showing hyperchromatic nuclei

Table 4-1. Comparative Cytomorphology of Thyroiditis

ABC	ACUTE THYROIDITIS	SUBACUTE THYROIDITIS	LYMPHOCYTIC THYROIDITIS	INVASIVE FIBROUS THYROIDITIS
Diathesis				
Colloid	−	±	±	−
Inflammatory cells	Neutrophils	Lymphocytes, mature	Lymphocytes, different maturation stages	Lymphocytes, few
Necrotic debris	+++	±	−	−
Follicular cells	±	±	++	−
Hürthle cells	−	−	++	−
Other cells	Macrophages	Epithelioid cells Multinucleated giant cells	−	Fibroblasts, rare

and abundant and peripheral vacuolated cytoplasm (Fig. 4-5). The intracytoplasmic vacuoles may contain colloid substance that stains pink with the MGG method. These "flare" cells are not specific for Graves disease since they may be seen in aspirates of a lymphocytic thyroiditis.

Nodular colloid goiter can be endemic or sporadic. It may mimic a thyroid tumor, and it is the most common thyroid lesion investigated by NAB in nonendemic areas. Aspirates from a well-established nodular colloid goiter reveal abundant colloid material and clusters and irregular large sheets of follicular cells with honeycomb pattern (Fig. 4-6A and B). The lesion may contain areas with Hürthle cell changes, harbor an autonomous toxic nodule, or undergo hemorrhagic degenerative changes. NAB from these foci may detect groups of Hürthle cells, clusters of vacuolated hyperplastic follicular cells, as seen in Graves disease, or numerous hemosiderin-laden macrophages, respectively.

Neoplasms

Follicular tumor. Follicular adenoma and follicular carcinoma of the thyroid are practically grouped under the large category of follicular tumor on cytologic bases since they yield in NAB strikingly similar cells. A diagnosis of follicular carcinoma can only be made when capsular or vascular invasion is demonstrated on careful histologic examination of the excised tumor.

Follicular adenoma has four histologic subtypes: colloid or macrofollicular, simple, microfollicular, and trabecular. ABC of a simple-type tumor is similar to that of normal thyroid tissue. A macrofollicular adenoma yields cellular material indistinguishable from the ABC of a colloid goiter. A microfollicular adenoma shows in NAB

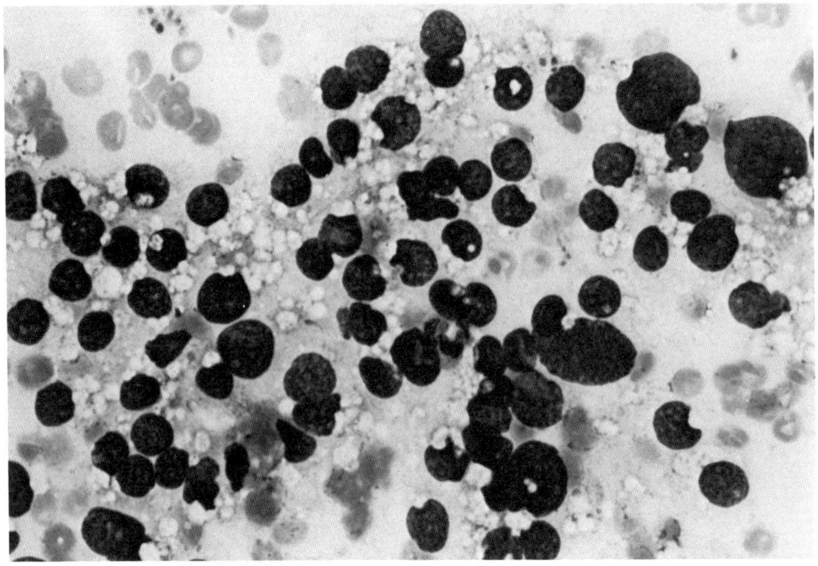

Figure 4-5. Graves' disease. A cluster of follicular cells with abundant and vacuolated cytoplasm and hyperchromatic pleomorphic nuclei. (MGG ×400.)

syncytial clusters of follicular cells in follicular grouping and little or no colloid material (Fig. 4-7). Individual tumor cells usually show regular and round nuclei without nucleoli. Prominent nucleoli may be seen in some cases. Trabecular adenoma shows in aspirates syncytial clusters of follicular cells with ground glass nuclei and intranuclear cytoplasmic inclusions, similar to those seen in papillary carcinoma of the thyroid.

Well-differentiated follicular carcinomas yield cellular material similar to that of follicular adenomas of the thyroid. Poorly differentiated follicular carcinomas, however, may show pleomorphic malignant cells in a follicular grouping.

Papillary carcinoma constitutes about 60% of all thyroid cancers. It has four histologic patterns: papillary, follicular, solid, and sclerosing. The main histologic criteria of this tumor are cytologic, namely, the presence of overlapping ground glass nuclei, nuclear grooves or ridges, and intranuclear cytoplasmic inclusions. These are applicable in the cytologic identification of the papillary carcinoma.

NAB from a papillary-type tumor reveals cells in large irregular, monolayered, and syncytial sheets with or without follicular arrangements. The tumor cells are usually cuboidal, but rarely columnar, squamoid, or spindle-shaped. Their nuclei are round or vesicular and display a finely granular chromatin pattern. Single or multiple nucleoli may be seen. Linear chromatin ridges or nuclear grooves and intranuclear cytoplasmic inclusions are commonly seen in abundance (Figs. 4-8 and 4-9). Psammoma bodies, ropy colloid strands, multinucleated giant cells, and numerous lymphoid cells may also be seen. Blood is a common background substance, and hemosiderin-laden macrophages may be seen.

The follicular variant of papillary carcinoma yields in NAB irregular syncytial clusters of tumor cells showing nuclear features similar to those of a classic papillary carcinoma (Fig. 4-10).

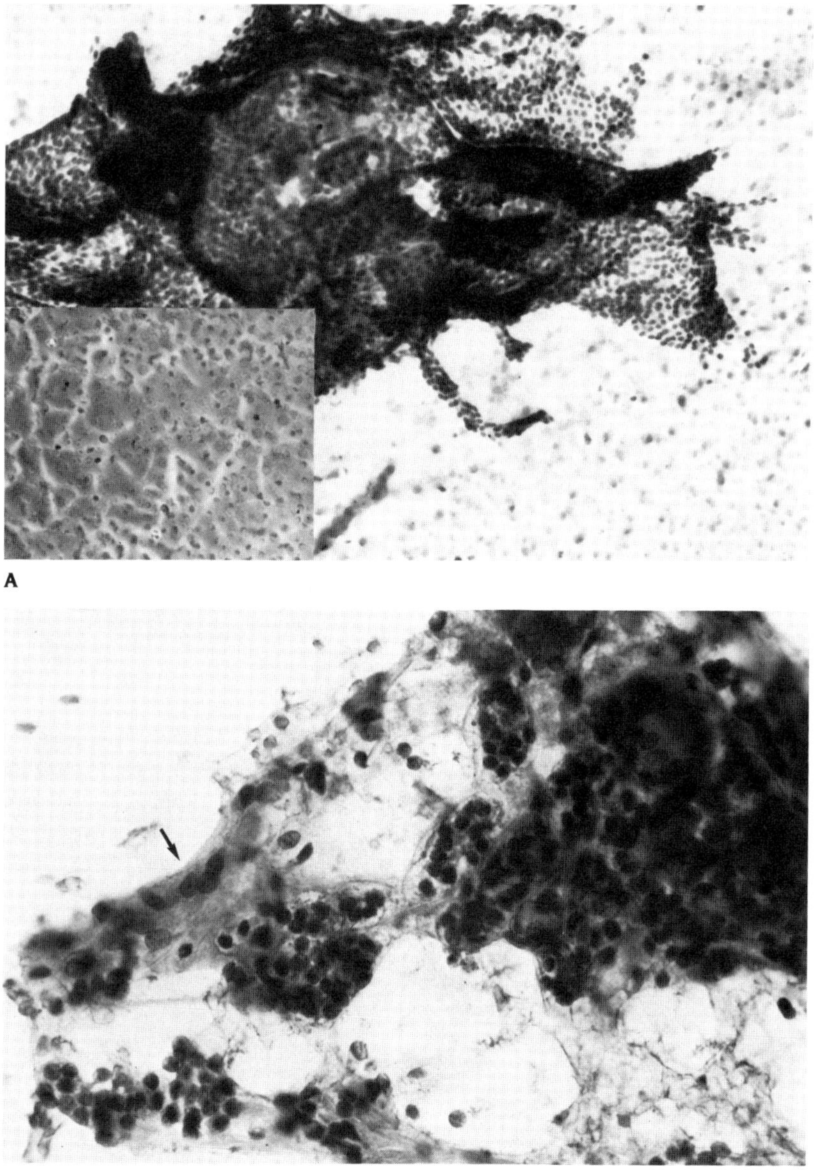

A

B

Figure 4-6. Nodular colloid goiter. **A.** A large branching fragment of follicular epithelium with folding in a granular colloid backgound. **Inset:** colloid material showing characteristic cracking pattern (MGG ×100; **Inset** ×40). **B.** Groups of follicular cells in colloid background. A thick colloid strand containing a few naked nuclei is noted (*arrow*). (Papanicolaou ×250.)

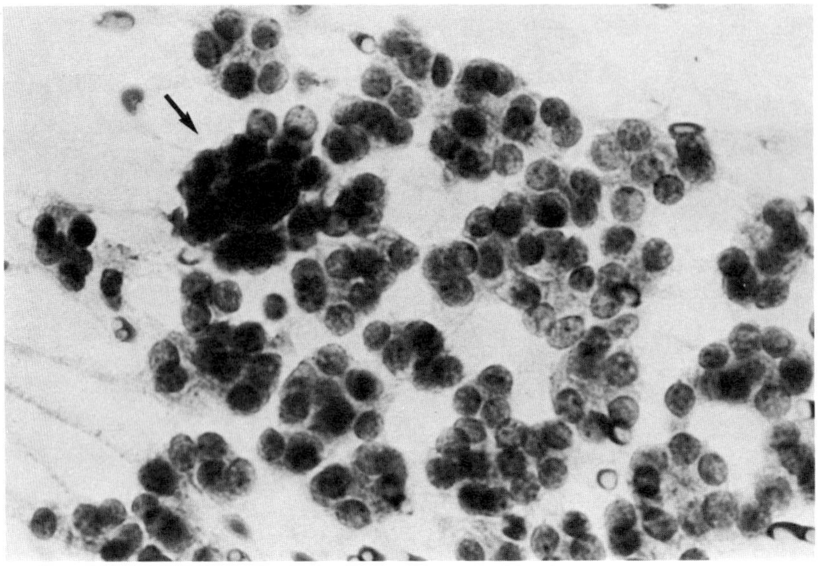

Figure 4-7. Follicular neoplasm showing benign-appearing follicular cells in syncytium with focal follicular formation containing colloid material (*arrow*). (Papanicolaou ×400.)

Hürthle cell tumor has been regarded as a malignant or a potentially malignant tumor of the thyroid. NAB from the tumor in most of the cases shows a monomorphic cell population consisting of single or loose groups of large, oval, or polygonal cells with granular eosinophilic cytoplasm. The nuclei are usually small, round, single, or double and eccentrically located. Macronucleoli may be present (Fig. 4-11).

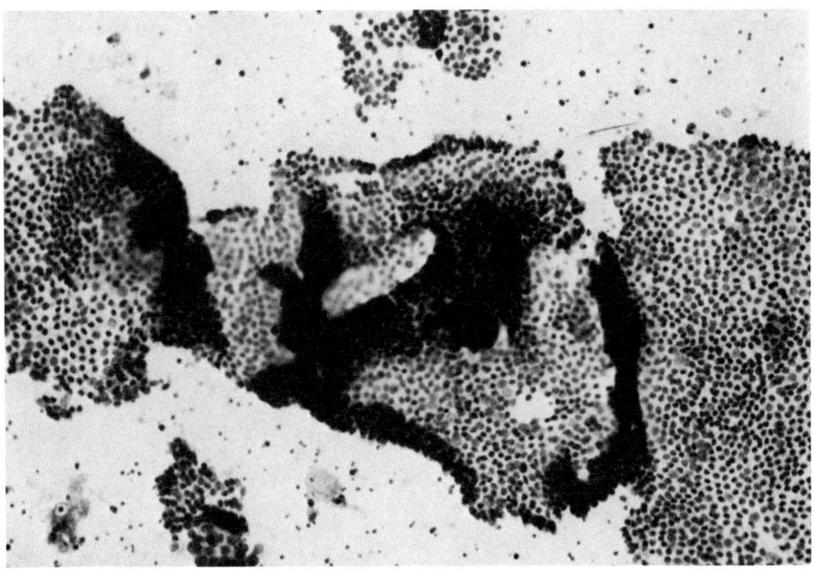

Figure 4-8. Papillary carcinoma showing irregular and large fragment of neoplastic epithelium. (Papanicolaou ×100.)

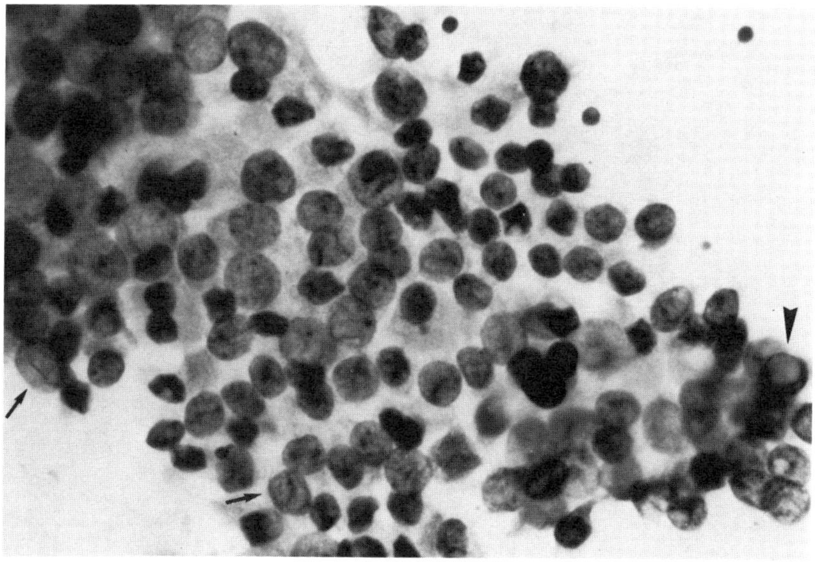

Figure 4-9. Papillary carcinoma. A syncytial fragment of tumor epithelium showing intranuclear cytoplasmic inclusions (*arrowhead*) and nuclear grooves (*arrow*). (Papanicolaou ×400.)

Medullary carcinoma. The majority of thyroid medullary carcinomas are sporadic, but about 15 to 30% of them may be associated with types II and III multiple endocrine neoplasia syndrome. Elevated serum calcitonin constitutes the most sensitive marker of the tumor. NAB from the tumor may reveal pleomorphic tumor cells that are polygonal, plasmacytoid, spindle-shaped, or small and round. They

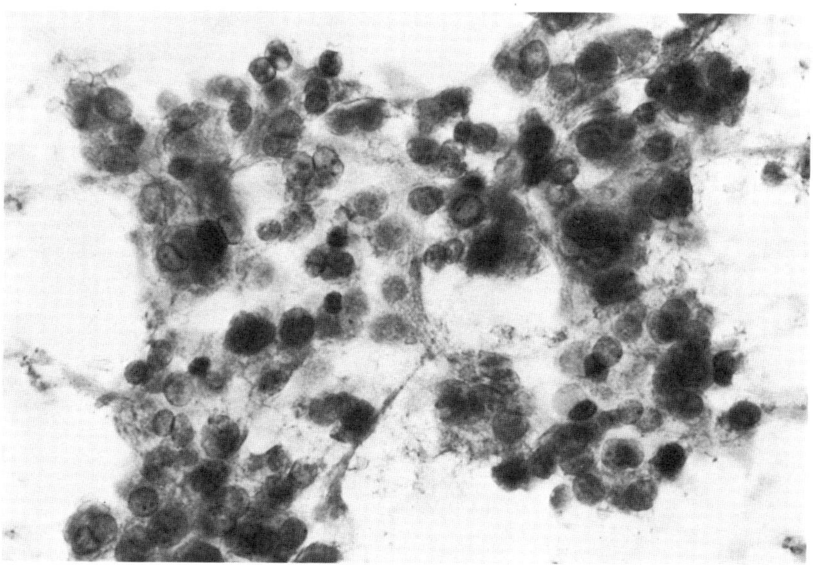

Figure 4-10. Papillary carcinoma, follicular variant, showing a syncytial fragment of tumor epithelium consisting of cells with intranuclear cytoplasmic inclusions. (Papanicolaou ×250.)

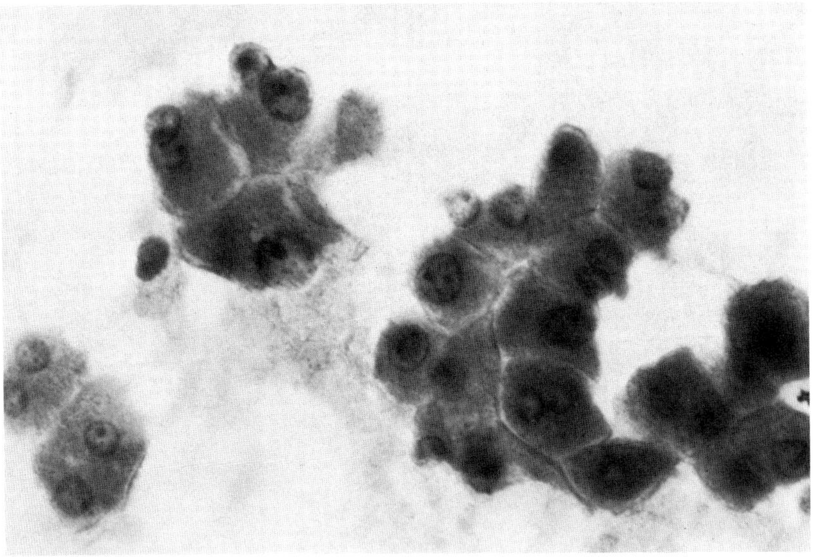

Figure 4-11. Hürthle cell tumor showing loose groups of large polygonal tumor cells with eccentrically located round nuclei containing macronucleoli and granular cytoplasm. (Papanicolaou ×400.)

present singly or in loosely cohesive clusters with syncytial grouping. The nuclei are round, oval, or multilobulated. Intracytoplasmic azurophil granules may be present. The smear background may contain amorphous and granular amyloid material (Figs. 4-12 and 4-13). Calcitonin granules, demonstrated by the immunoperoxidase

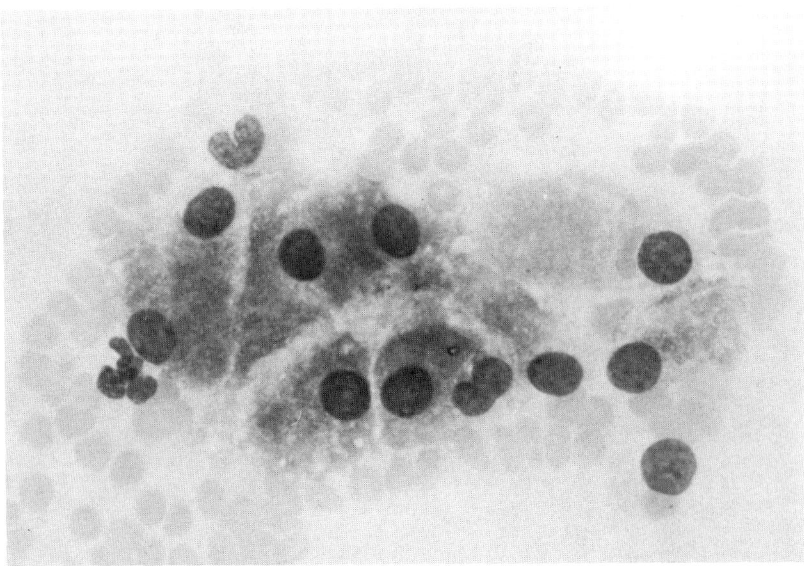

Figure 4-12. Medullary carcinoma. Large and pleomorphic tumor cells with intracytoplasmic azurophil granules. (MGG ×400.)

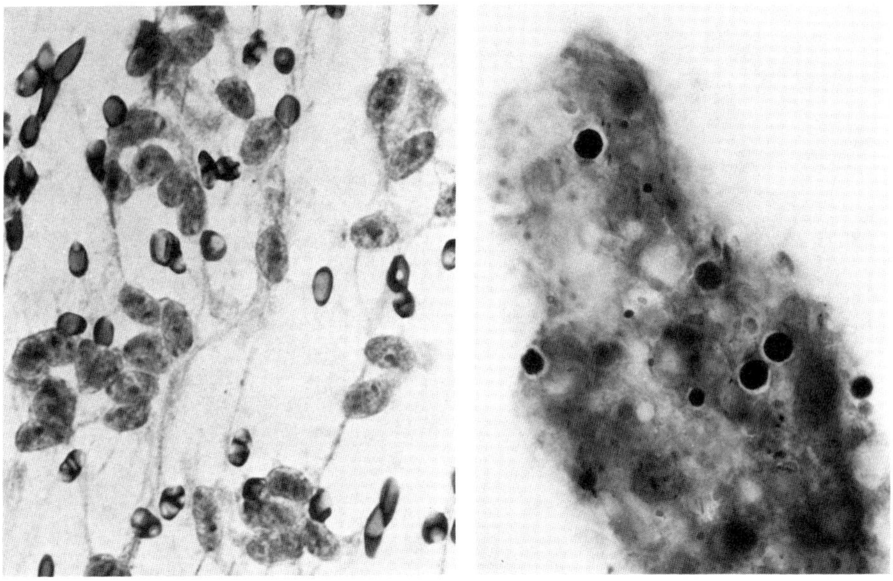

A B

Figure 4-13. Medullary carcinoma. **A.** Dyshesive and loose clusters of small tumor cells with vesicular and spindle-shaped nuclei. **B.** Amyloid material containing calcified bodies. (Papanicolaou, **A** ×400, **B** ×100.)

technique, applied directly to the Papanicolaou stain slide, are diagnostic of the tumor.

Anaplastic carcinoma is highly aggressive and rarely occurs in patients under 60 years of age. The tumor may be composed of small malignant cells, spindle-shaped cells, or giant cells, with or without a squamous cell component. The majority of so-called small cell anaplastic cancers of the thyroid are actually lymphomas when further studied. NAB from an anaplastic thyroid carcinoma reveals pleomorphic malignant cells with single or multiple macronucleoli. The smear background contains necrotic debris and numerous polymorphonuclear leukocytes (Fig. 4-14).

Cellular features of four major types of thyroid carcinoma are summarized in Table 4-2.

Other thyroid cancers. Metastatic carcinomas to the thyroid are found in about 10% of patients with cancers arising elsewhere in the body. The most common primary tumors are cutaneous melanoma and carcinomas of the breast, lung, and kidney.

Primary non-Hodgkin's lymphomas are found mainly in elderly patients who had lymphocytic thyroiditis. Hodgkin's disease primarily involving the thyroid is extremely rare.

Thyroid cancers in children. All types of thyroid carcinoma in adults are found in children. Among these papillary carcinomas are the commonest, and about 40% of them arise in thyroid affected by lymphocytic thyroiditis.

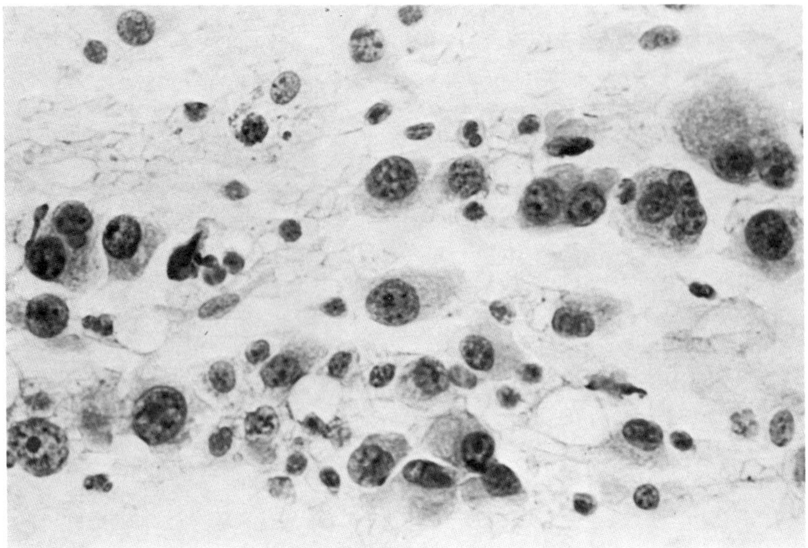

Figure 4-14. Anaplastic carcinoma showing large pleomorphic malignant cells with marconucleoli. (Papanicolaou X250.)

Diagnostic Accuracy

The thyroid is a highly vascularized organ. Therefore, a biopsy needle larger than 22-gauge is contraindicated. The aspirated cellular material is usually diluted with blood, and to obtain a cellular smear, excessive liquid blood should be drained off the slide prior to smear preparation. One of the most important prerequisites for an accurate cytodiagnosis of thyroid lesions is an adequate and representative cell sample. Criteria for an adequate cell sample are subjective. In Kini's experience about 20% of all thyroid aspirates were inadequate for cytologic evaluation; for a confident cytodiagnosis she required six smears prepared from six different sites of each given thyroid nodule with at least six to eight clusters of follicular cells on every two smears. Goellner considered a sample adequate if it contained 5 to 6 groups of well-preserved follicular cells with 10 or more cells in each group. In our experience an adequate specimen consists of a total of at least 10 large clusters of follicular cells containing more than 20 cells present on all available smears.

As a screening procedure for thyroid tumor detection, NAB has proved to be reliable. Frable and Frable analyzed nine series of thyroid NAB, including their own, and concluded that an overall positive predictive value (presence of disease) was within the 89 to 95% range, and a negative predictive value (absence of disease) was within the 93.6 to 99.3% range for solitary thyroid nodules, with 20% of them neoplastic in nature.

In a recent review of 24 large series of NAB of solitary thyroid nodules, adequate cell samples between 70 and 98% (mean 88.2%) had been obtained. An overall diagnostic accuracy between 60 and 100% (mean 91.1%), a false-negative rate of 0 to 27.5% (mean 8.8%), and a false-positive rate of 0 to 40% (mean 6.7%) were observed. In a series which follicular neoplasms were excluded from the statistical analysis, the false-positive rate was reduced to 2%.

Table 4-2. Cytomorphology of Thyroid Neoplasms

ABC	FOLLICULAR NEOPLASM	PAPILLARY CARCINOMA	HÜRTHLE CELL TUMOR	MEDULLARY CARCINOMA	ANAPLASTIC CARCINOMA
Diathesis					
Colloid	±	±(MGG)	±	±	–
Other	–	Lymphoid cells	–	Amyloid	Necrotic debris Neutrophils
Tumor cells					
Arrangement	Syncytia or acini containing colloid	Papillary fronds Sheets	Single Dyshesive clusters	Single Dyshesive clusters	Single
Shape	Polygonal	Polygonal	Polygonal	Pleomorphic Spindle Plasmacytoid	Pleomorphic
Cytoplasm	Ill-defined, scant	Ill-defined, scant	Well-defined, abundant	Variable Azurophil granules (MGG)	Well-defined
Nuclei	Round Pleomorphic	Vesicular	Round Pleomorphic	Round Pleomorphic	Pleomorphic
Macronucleoli	±	±	±	+	+
Nuclear inclusions and grooves	±	+++	+++	±	±

In experienced hands the cytodiagnosis of thyroid cancers has a high diagnostic accuracy: 90 to 98% for papillary carcinomas, 85 to 90% for Hürthle cell tumors, and 80% for medullary carcinomas.

Diagnostic Pitfalls

Cytodiagnostic pitfalls may be encountered in all kinds of thyroid lesion, whether they are inflammatory or neoplastic in nature. On some occasions, two lesions may coexist in one diseased thyroid, making the cytologic diagnosis very difficult.

Thyroiditis vs. thyroid neoplasm. The cytodiagnosis of thyroiditis is usually straightforward, especially when clinical, biochemical, and serological data are taken into consideration. Diagnostic traps occur mainly with Hashimoto's disease showing bizarre Hürthle cells that are usually seen in cohesive clusters. They show bland nuclei without prominent nucleoli generally. On rare occasions, Hashimoto's thyroiditis may harbor a Hürthle cell tumor, papillary carcinoma, or non-Hodgkin's lymphoma that yields in NAB characteristic cells in addition to those of a lymphocytic thyroiditis.

Nodular colloid goiter vs. thyroid neoplasm. The cytodiagnosis of nodular colloid goiter is usually not difficult. NAB from a cellular area with hyperplastic follicular cells or Hürthle cells may pose differential diagnostic problems with a follicular neoplasm or a Hürthle cell tumor. This problem can be practically solved by having cell samples taken from different areas of the nodular colloid goiter; consequently, the cellular features of colloid goiter predominate in the additional samples. It is important to note that aspirates from a nodular colloid goiter, toxic diffuse goiter, and follicular neoplasms of the thyroid usually show numerous naked nuclei that do not seem to have any diagnostic value for these lesions.

Thyroid neoplasms. The cytodiagnosis of papillary carcinoma in typical cases is not difficult. A false-negative diagnosis is usually due to inadequate sampling. It is important to note that cystic degenerative changes occur in about 10% of all papillary carcinomas. Thus, a careful search for sheets of cells showing nuclei with a powdery chromatin pattern, intranuclear cytoplasmic inclusions, and nuclear grooves should be done in all cyst contents to rule out or confirm the possibility of a papillary carcinoma. These nuclear characteristics must be present in abundance to have a diagnostic value for papillary carcinoma. Intranuclear cytoplasmic inclusions occasionally are seen in cells aspirated from other types of thyroid tumors.

Cells aspirated from a thyroid medullary carcinoma may be mistaken for those of a Hürthle cell tumor, papillary carcinoma, or anaplastic carcinoma of the gland. However, medullary carcinoma cells are more pleomorphic and stain positively with calcitonin antiserum, and amyloid material may be present on the smear background. Electron microscopic study of aspirated tumor cells of medullary carcinoma reveals intracytoplasmic neurosecretory-type granules.

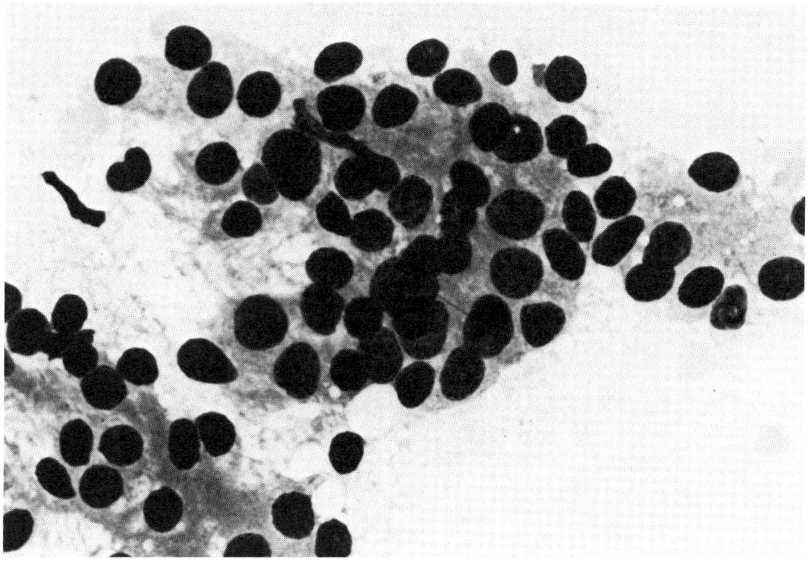

Figure 4-15. Parathyroid adenoma showing clustered tumor cells with abundant granular cytoplasm. (Diff-Quik ×400.)

The diagnosis of a thyroid anaplastic carcinoma should be easy in a representative cell sample. It is important to reemphasize that thyroid anaplastic carcinoma is an aggressive and rapidly growing tumor that commonly undergoes extensive necrosis. Therefore, necrotic and purulent material aspirated from a thyroid mass may represent only the necrotic part of an anaplastic carcinoma. A diligent search for malignant cells in these specimens, and NAB of any palpable residual nodule should always be done.

PARATHYROID

Mass lesions of the parathyroids include cyst, adenoma, and carcinoma of the glands. They are rare targets of NAB.

Parathyroid cysts are usually nonfunctioning and arise from the inferior glands. NAB of these cysts often reveals a variable amount of a clear fluid, which is usually scanty in cellularity. A specific diagnosis of a parathyroid cyst may be made if parathyroid tissue is histologically identified in the excised cyst wall, or if the cyst content shows an elevated level of parathyroid hormone.

Parathyroid adenoma and carcinoma are classically associated with hyperparathyroidism. NAB from these lesions reveals clusters of epithelial cells with ill-defined abundant cytoplasm and round nuclei. They resemble thyroid follicular cells. Nuclear pleomorphism and conspicuous nucleoli may be seen in both adenoma and carcinoma of the glands, and the cytologic distinction between these two lesions is almost impossible by means of ABC (Fig. 4-15).

SUGGESTED READING

Frable WJ, Frable MA: Fine needle aspiration biopsy of the thyroid. Histopathologic and clinical considerations. In Fenoglio C and Wolff M: *Progress in Surgical Pathology*. New York, Saunders, 1983, Vol 1 pp 152–181.

Goellner JR, Gharib H, Grant CS, et al.: Fine needle aspiration cytology of the thyroid, 1980–1986. *Acta Cytol* 1987;31:587–590.

Goellner JR, Carney JA: Cytologic features of fine needle aspirates of hyalinizing trabecular adenoma of the thyroid. *Am J Clin Pathol* 1989;91:115–119.

Kini SR, Miller JM, Hamburger SI, et al.: Cytopathology of follicular lesions of the thyroid gland. *Diagn Cytopathol* 1985;1:123–132.

Kini SR: *Guides to Clinical Aspiration Biopsy: Thyroid*. New York, Igaku-Shoin, 1987.

Lowhagen T, Linsk JA: Aspiration biopsy cytology of the thyroid gland. In Linsk JA, Franzen S: *Clinical Aspiration Cytology*, ed 2. Philadelphia, Lippincott, 1989, pp 61–90.

Nathan AR, Raines KB, Lee M Y-T, et al.: Fine needle aspiration biopsy of cold thyroid nodules. *Cancer* 1988;62:1337–1342.

Nguyen GK, Ginsberg J. Crockford PM: Fine needle aspiration biopsy of the thyroid. Its value and limitations in the diagnosis and management of solitary thyroid nodules. *Pathol Annu*, (part I) 1991;25:63–91.

Rupp M, Ehya H: Nuclear grooves in the aspiration cytology of papillary carcinoma of the thyroid. *Acta Cytol* 1989;33:21–26.

5

SALIVARY GLANDS AND OTHER NECK MASSES

The exact nature of masses arising in the vicinity of the salivary glands cannot be determined with certainty by means of physical examination, biochemical tests, and radiologic imaging techniques. NAB has proved to be the most economical and reliable method of obtaining morphologic diagnoses of these lesions.

INDICATIONS AND CONTRAINDICATIONS FOR NAB

Any mass lesions of the head and neck, including salivary glands, are targets of NAB. This technique of investigation is contraindicated in patients with bleeding disorders and in those who are suspected to have a carotid body tumor, as needling of this neoplasm may cause severe bleeding and thrombosis of the carotid arteries. Preoperative knowledge of the benign or malignant nature of a salivary gland mass helps the surgeon to plan the extent of the surgical intervention. The NAB in most situations can be helpful in determining the origin of a neck mass since a branchial

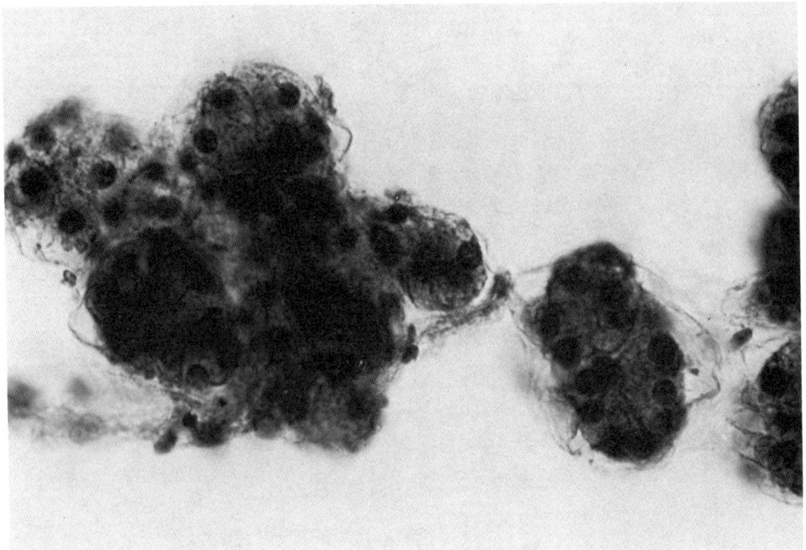

Figure 5-1. Normal salivary gland. Lobules of serous acini. (Papanicolaou ×250.)

cleft cyst, a carotid body tumor, or an enlarged lymph node located adjacent to a salivary gland may mimic a tumor of the gland clinically.

SALIVARY GLANDS

Normal cellular elements of a salivary gland are commonly seen in needle aspirates from the gland. Excretory ducts appear as flat sheets or clusters of cuboidal or columnar cells with scanty cytoplasm and round or oval nuclei. Acinar cells are seen in clusters or as ball-like structures with round and basally located nuclei. Their cytoplasm is clear, vacuolated, or finely granular, depending on the mucous or serous type of gland (Fig. 5-1). Spindle-shaped myoepithelial cells may also be seen.

Benign Nonneoplastic Lesions

Mucocele or retention cyst usually occurs as the result of an obstruction of the excretory duct of a minor salivary gland. It is seen mainly in two locations: the lower lip and mouth floor. The lesion is almost always evident clinically, and it rarely is a target of NAB. Aspirate from a mucocele reveals mucus, a few inflammatory cells, and degenerated epithelial cells.

Acute sialadenitis is caused by bacterial or viral infection. It is usually evident clinically and does not need morphologic confirmation by NAB.

Chronic nonspecific sialadenitis often results from an obstruction of the excretory duct of a major salivary gland by a calculus. NAB from the inflamed gland shows benign glandular cells, lymphoid cells, and plasma cells. Metaplastic squamous cells may also be seen.

Benign lymphoepithelial lesion of major salivary glands may occur as part of Sjögren's syndrome. It also may be associated with or precede a disseminated lymphoma. ABC of a such lesion is similar to that of a chronic nonspecific sialadenitis. However, lymphoid cells are much more abundant. When a lymphoma is suspected by ABC, the involved gland should be excised for histologic study.

Benign Tumors

Pleomorphic adenomas (mixed tumors) constitute about 75% of all salivary gland tumors. The majority of these neoplasms arise from the parotid glands. Histologically, they are characterized by a mixture of benign epithelial and stromal elements in different proportions. The epithelial cells are glandular in type and may show oncocytic or squamous metaplastic changes. The stroma is usually myxomatous and contains round or stellate cells. Areas of cartilaginous tissue and hyaline connective tissue may be present. The ABC of pleomorphic adenomas correlates well with their histologic patterns. Aspirates are usually cell-rich and show a myxoid background. There are isolated stellate cells and tight clusters of benign epithelial cells. Additionally, there may be fragments of myxomatous stromal tissue composed of stellate cells as well as cells with transitional features between epithelial and stromal cells, squamous cells, and oncocytes (Figs. 5-2 to 5-4). When atypical-appearing tumor cells are seen, the excised lesion should be examined extensively to rule out evidence of an invasive malignant mixed tumor.

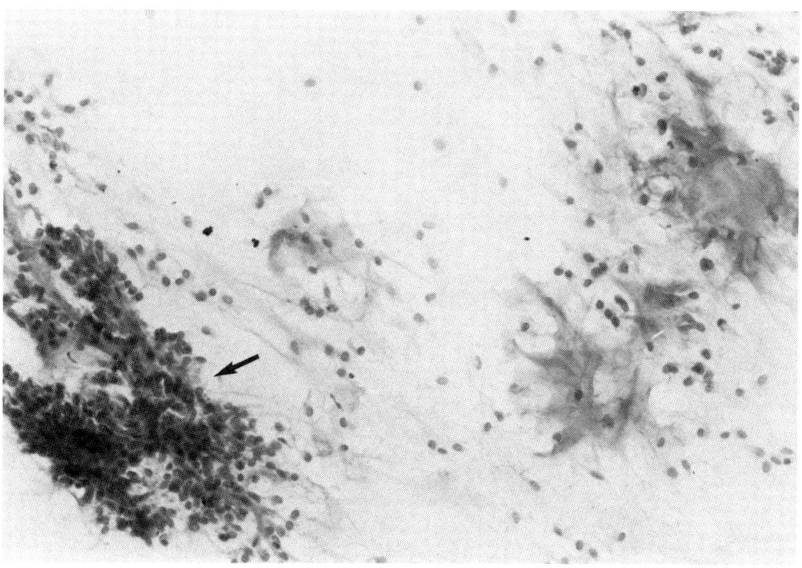

Figure 5-2. Pleomorphic adenoma. Low-power view reveals myxoid background containing stellate cells and a large irregular group of epithelial cells (*arrow*). (Papanicolaou ×100.)

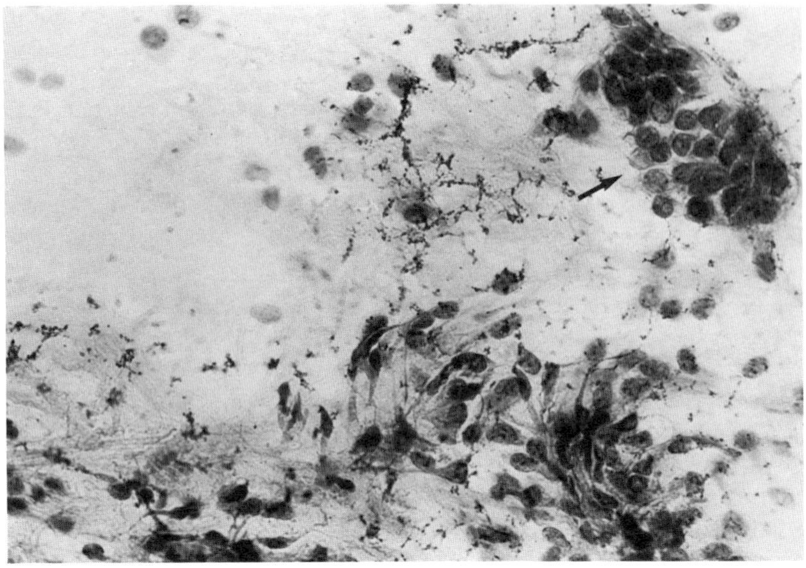

Figure 5-3. Pleomorphic adenoma. A fragment of benign glandular epithelium (*arrow*) and an irregular fragment of myxomatous stroma containing stellate cells. (Papanicolaou ×400.)

Monomorphic adenomas consist of several histologic variants such as adenolymphoma (Warthin tumor), oxyphilic adenoma, basal cell adenoma, and sebaceous adenoma. Of these, adenolymphomas are the commonest and constitute approximately 20% of all salivary gland tumors. They usually occur in the parotid glands and may be solid or cystic. NAB from an adenolymphoma yields three

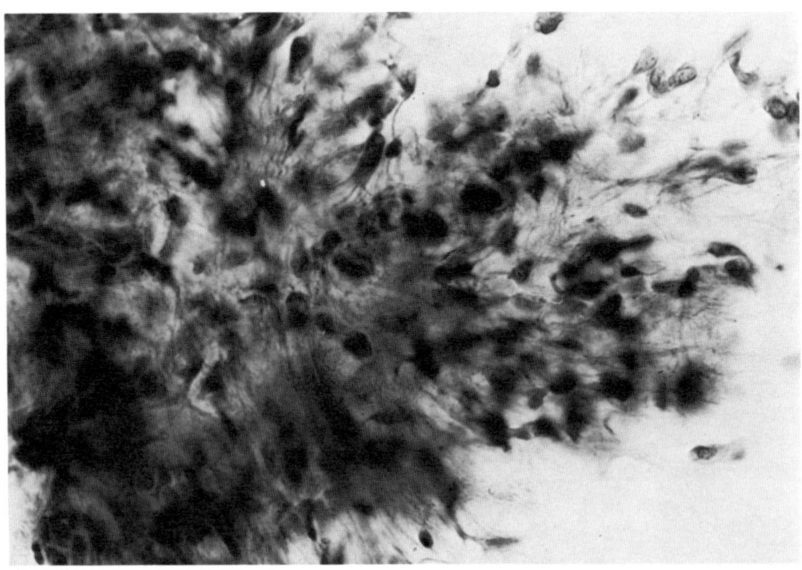

Figure 5-4. Pleomorphic adenoma. An irregular fragment of connective tissue containing stellate cells. (Papanicolaou ×250.)

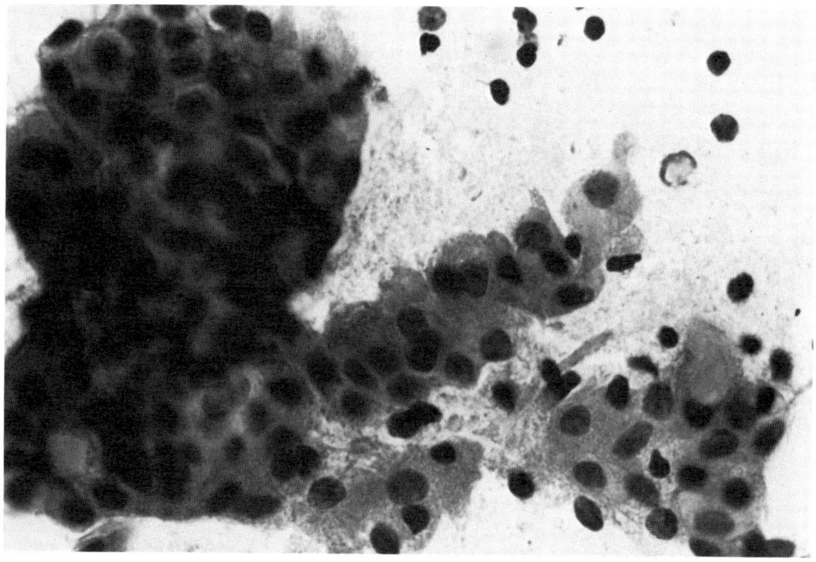

Figure 5-5. Adenolymphoma. Sheets of oncocytic epithelium and benign lymphoid cells. Note background debris. (Papanicolaou ×250.)

cellular components in variable amounts: lymphocytes, oncocytes, and oncocytic ghost cells. The oncocytes are generally in monolayered sheets but may be double layered, picket fence style, or isolated (Fig. 5-5.)

Malignant Tumors

Mucoepidermoid carcinomas are the most common cancers of the salivary glands. They are classified as low-grade and high-grade tumors. Low-grade mucoepidermoid carcinomas are composed of mucus-secreting cells and malignant squamous cells showing a mild degree of dedifferentiation. High-grade tumors are characterized by highly malignant squamous cells, with some showing mucous secretion. ABC of a low-grade mucoepidermoid carcinoma reveals clusters of malignant squamous cells mixed with benign-appearing mucus-secreting cells (Fig. 5-6). A high-grade tumor yields mainly pleomorphic malignant squamous cells. Mucus-secreting cells may be of the squamous metaplastic variety, and the mucus is difficult to identify without a mucicarmine stain.

Adenoid cystic carcinomas are uncommon and usually occur in submandibular glands. Histologically, the tumors are characterized by small cuboidal cells arranged in anastomotic cordons and sheets, or around cystic spaces containing homogenous or fibrillary material. The stroma may be markedly hyalinized. The ABC of adenoid cystic carcinoma reveals small, regular, basaloid cells present singly, in irregular sheets, or as spherical clusters containing amorphous (hyalinized) core material. These classic spherical structures are rounded and slightly basophilic (Fig. 5-7).

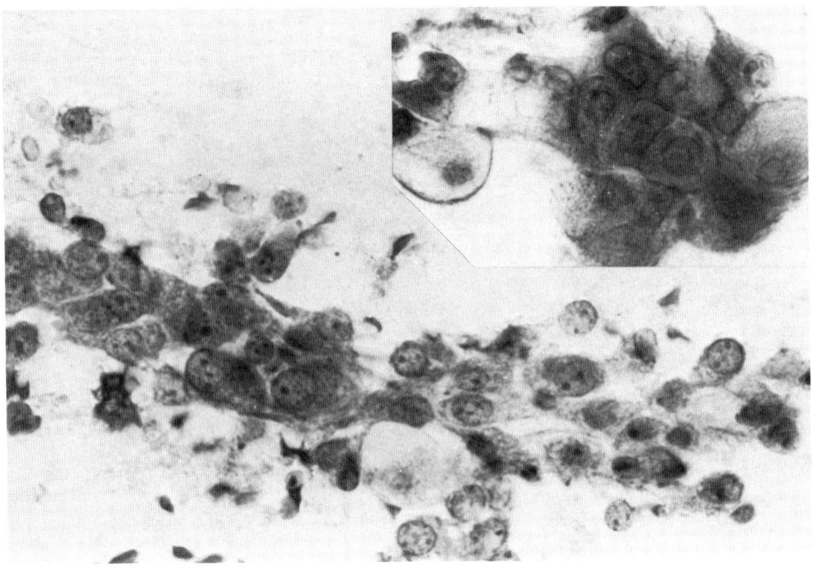

Figure 5-6. Low-grade mucoepidermoid carcinoma. Irregular fragments of malignant squamous epithelium and a few benign-appearing mucus-secreting cells. **Inset:** A few mucus-secreting cells and malignant squamous cells. (Papanicolaou ×400.)

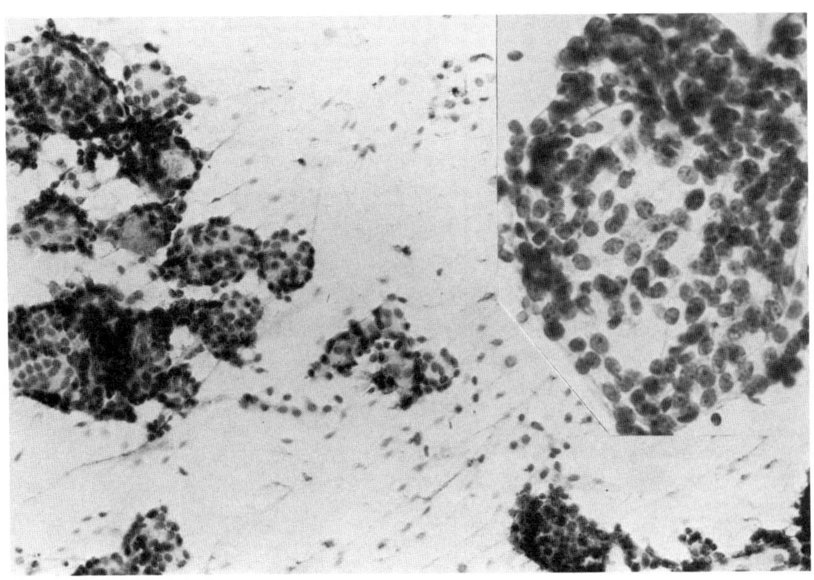

Figure 5-7. Adenoid cystic carcinoma. Characteristic ball-like clusters of tumor cells with hyaline globules. **Inset:** A ball of tumor cells. (Papanicolaou ×100, **Inset** ×250).

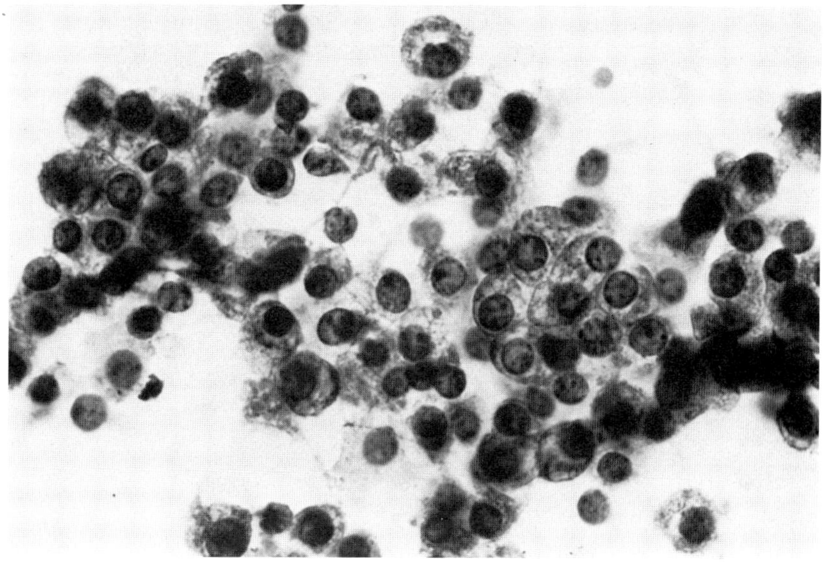

Figure 5-8. Acinic cell carcinoma. Sheets and clusters of rounded tumor cells showing abundant granular or vacuolated cytoplasm. (Papanicolaou ×400.)

Acinic cell carcinomas are rare and occur predominantly in parotid glands. Histologically, they are usually solid and composed of uniform tumor cells arranged in cords and acini separated by scant stroma. The tumor cells are polygonal with abundant, clear, or granular cytoplasm, and small and vesicular nuclei showing inconspicuous nucleoli. The aspirate shows numerous tumor cells singly, in clusters, and in monolayered sheets. There also may be naked nuclei. The moderate-sized cells show abundant, clear, or granular cytoplasm and round or vesicular bland nuclei (Fig. 5-8).

Malignant pleomorphic adenomas may arise de novo or from a preexisting pleomorphic adenoma. In the former situation, both malignant epithelial and stromal cells are seen in the tumor aspirates. In the latter case, malignant squamous and glandular cells or basaloid cells are seen, as well as benign cellular elements of a pleomorphic adenoma.

Other cancers of the salivary glands, such as squamous carcinoma, adenocarcinoma, undifferentiated large and small cell carcinomas, Hodgkin's disease, and non-Hodgkin's lymphoma, are rare occurrences. Metastatic carcinomas from the breast, kidney, lung, and melanoma are occasionally encountered in the salivary glands. These aspirates are comparable to those of tumors arising from other sites described elsewhere.

Cellular features of some commonly encountered tumors of the salivary glands are summarized in Table 5-1.

Table 5-1. Comparative Cytology of Salivary Gland Tumors

TUMOR TYPES	CYSTIC CHANGES	MUCINOUS MATERIAL	LYMPHOCYTES	TUMOR CELLS	OTHER FINDINGS
Pleomorphic adenoma	–	+	–	Epithelial-cell clusters Mesenchymal cells, single and clustered	
Adenolymphoma	±	–	+++	Oncocytes	Ghost cells Debris
Mucoepidermoid tumor					
Low-grade	+	+	–	Squamous and mucous cells	
High-grade	–	±	–	Pleomorphic squamous and glandular cells	
Adenoid cystic carcinoma	±	±	–	Basaloid cells in balls and sheets	Mucoid spherical bodies
Acinic cell carcinoma	±	–	±	Polygonal cells in sheets and papillae	Naked nuclei
Malignant pleomorphic adenoma	–	±	–	Bizarre cells	Long standing tumor history

BRANCHIAL CLEFT CYST

This cyst occurs anterior to the sternocleidomastoid muscle and on the middle third of the neck. A noninfected cyst yields in NAB a few milliliters of a turbid fluid containing mature squamous cells and lymphoid cells. (Fig. 5-9). Glandular cells may also be present. Crystalline material and debris are background substances. Squamous cells with nuclear atypia may be seen in cases of infected branchial cleft cyst.

CAROTID BODY TUMOR

This extraadrenal paraganglioma is a slow-growing tumor. It yields in NAB numerous tumor cells present singly, in loose clusters, in rosettes, or in cell balls. They show ill-defined and granular cytoplasm, as well as slightly pleomorphic ovoid

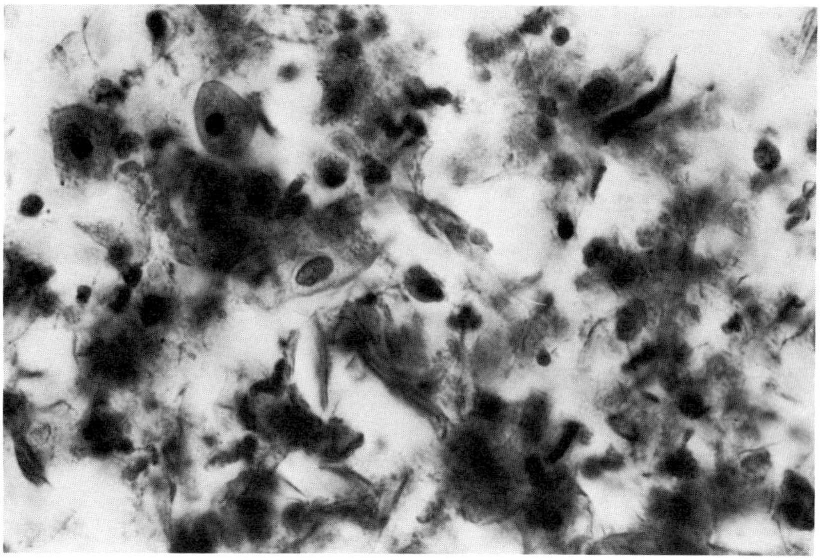

Figure 5-9. Branchial cleft cyst. Benign squamous cells mixed with inflammatory cells and background debris. (Papanicolaou X250.)

nuclei (Fig. 5-10). Their cytoplasm stains positively with neuron-specific enolase antiserum. Intracytoplasmic neurosecretory-type granules can be demonstrated by electron microscopic study of aspirated tumor cells.

DIAGNOSTIC ACCURACY

The cytodiagnostic accuracy of salivary gland tumors varies with their histologic types. In experienced hands, pleomorphic adenomas and acinic cell carcinomas may be correctly diagnosed by ABC in about 90% of the cases. However, the diagnostic accuracy is about 80% with mucoepidermoid carcinomas, 75% with adenolymphomas, 70% with adenoid cystic carcinomas, and 50% of cancers arising from a preexisting pleomorphic adenoma. It should be borne in mind that cytologic interpretation of salivary gland tumors is fraught with hazards, and histologic variations present in most tumors complicate the cytologic typing of salivary gland tumors.

DIAGNOSTIC PITFALLS

False-negative results are mainly encountered in cases of tumor with marked cystic degenerative changes, such as adenolymphomas and mucoepidermoid carcinomas that may yield in NAB only nondiagnostic cystic contents with no well-preserved tumor cells. Therefore, all palpable residual masses detected after evacuation of cystic contents must be aspirated for further cytologic evaluation.

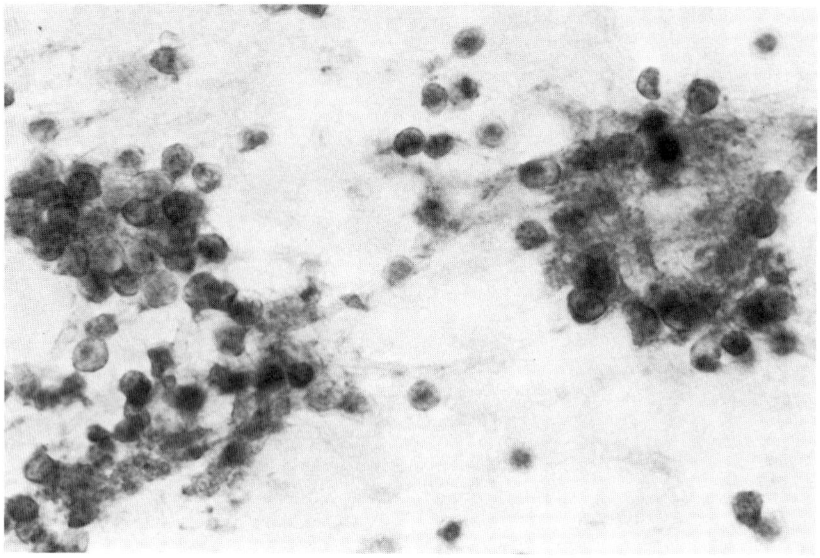

Figure 5-10. Carotid body tumor. Clusters of tumor cells showing ill-defined fibrillary cytoplasm. (Papanicolaou ×400.)

False-positive diagnoses may occur in cases of pleomorphic adenoma containing bizarre-looking epithelial elements. In this situation multiple sections of the excised tumor should be examined to rule out evidence of an invasion seen in a malignant pleomorphic adenoma. Degenerated oncocytes may be mistaken for malignant squamous cells. Cells of a cutaneous eccrine poroma or a basal cell adenoma of a salivary gland may mimic those of an adenoid cystic carcinoma. In this case the presence of mucoid globules and prominent nucleoli in tumor cell nuclei indicate an adenoid cystic carcinoma.

SUGGESTED READING

Eneroth CM, Zajicek J: Aspiration biopsy of salivary gland tumors. II. Morphologic studies on smears and histologic sections from oncocytic tumors: 45 cases of papillary cystadenoma lymphomatosum and 4 cases of oncocytoma. *Acta Cytol* 1965;9:355–361.

Eneroth CM, Zajicek J: Aspiration biopsy of salivary gland tumors. III. Morphologic studies on smears and histologic sections from 368 mixed tumors. *Acta Cytol* 1966;10:440–454.

Eneroth CM, Zajicek J: Aspiration biopsy of salivary gland tumors. IV. Morphologic studies on smears and histologic sections from 45 cases of adenoid cystic carcinoma. *Acta Cytol* 1969;13:59–63.

Eneroth CM, Jakobsson P, Zajicek J: Aspiration biopsy of salivary gland tumors. V. Morphologic investigations on smears and histologic sections of acinic cell carcinoma. *Acta Radiol* (*Suppl*) 1971;310:85–93.

Hood IC, Qizilbash AH, Young JEM: Fine needle aspiration biopsy of paragangliomas. Cytologic, light microscopic, and ultrastructural studies of 3 cases. *Acta Cytol* 1983;27:651–657.

Kline TS: Salivary glands. In *Handbook of Fine Needle Aspiration Biopsy Cytology*, ed 2. New York, Churchill Livingstone, 1988, pp 121–152.

Koss LG, Woyke S, Olszewski W: The salivary glands. In *Aspiration Biopsy Cytology. Cytologic Interpretation and Histologic Bases*. New York, Igaku-Shoin, 1984, pp 191–222.

Layfield LJ, Tan P, Glasgow BJ: Fine needle aspiration of salivary gland lesions. *Arch Pathol Lab Med* 1987;111:346–353.

Qizilbash AH, Young JEM: *Guides to Clinical Aspiration Biopsy. Head and Neck*. New York, Igaku-Shoin, 1988.

Zajicek J, Eneroth CM, Jakobsson P: Aspiration biopsy of salivary gland tumors. VI. Morphologic studies on smears and histologic sections from mucoepidermoid carcinoma. *Acta Cytol* 1976;20:35–41.

6

LYMPH NODES

Needle aspiration biopsy for cytologic evaluation of superficially and deeply located enlarged lymph nodes is a reliable and economical diagnostic procedure. Palpable lymph nodes can be safely aspirated after manual fixation of the overlying skin. Mediastinal, intraabdominal, retroperitoneal, and pelvic nonpalpable lymph nodes can undergo biopsy under guidance of radiologic imaging techniques such as ultrasonography, computed tomography, and fluoroscopy. The last method requires opacification of the lymph glands biopsied by lymphangiography. An enlarged mediastinal lymph node compressing the tracheobronchial tree may be safely aspirated under direct vision via a bronchoscope. Smears prepared from aspirated material may be fixed in 95% ethanol and stained by the Papanicolaou technique, by hematoxylin and eosin, and by other special staining procedures. They can be air-dried and stained by the May-Grünwald-Giemsa, Wright, or Diff-Quick methods. Air-dried material is particularly helpful in the cytodiagnosis of lymphoproliferative disorders.

INDICATIONS AND CONTRAINDICATIONS FOR NAB

NAB is indicated in patients who have enlarged lymph nodes of unknown etiology. The procedure is useful for confirming or ruling out the possibility of a malignant process involving the enlarged glands. It is also used to evaluate the extent of a known lymphoma above or below the diaphragm, to diagnose its recurrence, and to stage a cancer of the genitourinary system.

There are no absolute contraindications for NAB of a superficially palpable lymph node. However, NAB of lymphadenopathies involving mediastinal, intraabdominal, pelvic, and retroperitoneal lymph nodes is contraindicated in patients with bleeding disorders and in those who are suspected of having an intrathoracic or intraabdominal hydatid cyst. Severe emphysema, pulmonary hypertension, and prior pneumonectomy constitute additional contraindications for NAB of mediastinal lymph nodes.

LYMPHADENITIS

Acute lymphadenitis is usually clinically evident and does not need morphologic confirmation by aspiration biopsy cytology (ABC) unless a culture for microbiological identification is required. NAB from an acute bacterial lymphadenitis reveals necrotic debris and inflammatory exudate.

Chronic lymphadenitis, or reactive hyperplasia of nodal tissues, is a common target of NAB. Histologically, hyperplastic lymph nodes may have different histologic patterns, such as follicular hyperplasia, sinus histiocytosis, diffuse lymphocytic hyperplasia, and diffuse immunoblastic hyperplasia. An accurate cytologic identification of these histologic variants is impossible and impractical. In general, hyperplastic lymph nodes yield in NAB cellular material consisting of lymphoid cells at different stages of development, plasma cells, polymorphonuclear leukocytes, and histiocytes which may contain tingible bodies (Fig. 6-1). Lymph nodes draining an area of chronic dermatitis also may contain melanin pigment-laden macrophages.

Granulomatous lymphadenitis may develop as a result of a tuberculous infection or sarcoidosis. NAB from such lesions shows multinucleated Langerhans-type giant cells and clusters of epithelioid cells characterized by carrot-shaped or bean-shaped

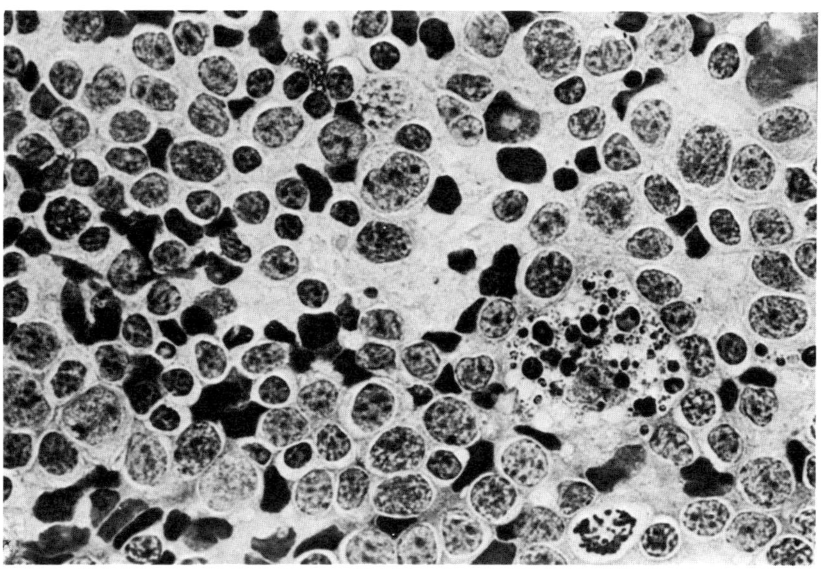

Figure 6-1. Hyperplastic lymph node. Lymphoid cells at different stages of maturation and a macrophage containing tingible bodies. (Papanicolaou ×500.)

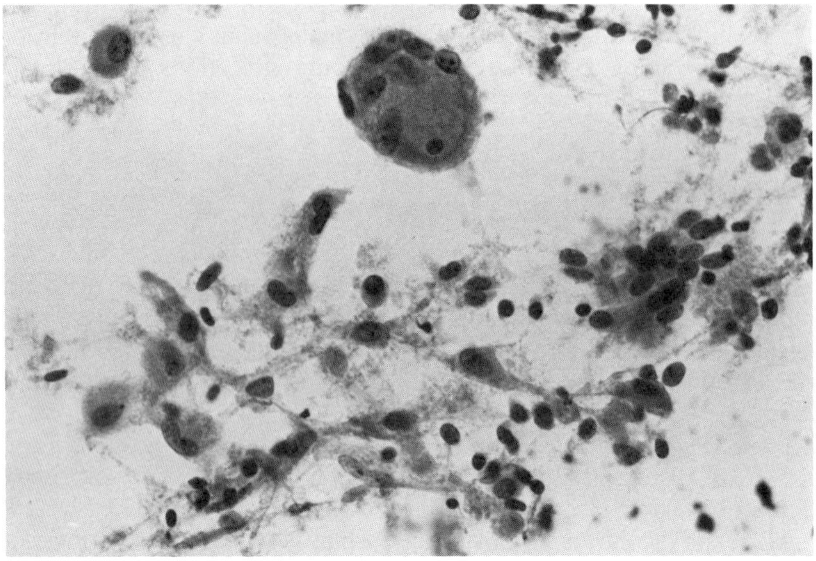

Figure 6-2. Tuberculous lymphadenitis. A multinucleated Langerhans giant cell, a few epithelioid cells, and necrotic material. (Papanicolaou ×250.)

nuclei and ill-defined cytoplasm (Fig. 6-2). Necrotic material is seen in cases of tuberculous lymphadenitis. Acid-fast bacilli may be visualized in Ziehl-Neelsen-stained smears. In sarcoidosis no necrotic material nor microorganisms are seen. However, multinucleated giant cells containing laminated Schaumann's bodies or star-shaped asteroid bodies may be present.

LYMPHOMA

Hodgkin's Lymphoma

Hodgkin's lymphoma can be classified into four histologic variants: lymphocytic predominance, nodular sclerosis, mixed cellularity, and lymphocytic depletion. The characteristic ABC pattern of Hodgkin's lymphoma is the presence of a polymorphic cell population containing lymphocytes; polymorphonuclear leukocytes, including eosinophils; histiocytes; and Reed-Sternberg cells. A cytodiagnosis of Hodgkin's lymphoma can only be made when Reed-Sternberg cells are clearly identified in the aspirate. These are large cells with abundant cytoplasm and a polylobed or bilobed nucleus containing an eosinophilic macronucleolus that occupies at least one-third of the nucleus. Not uncommonly, Hodgkin cells are also seen. They are large mononucleated cells (15 to 40 μm in diameter) showing a macronucleolus (Fig. 6-3). Usually, subclassification of Hodgkin's lymphoma is not possible by means of ABC.

Non-Hodgkin's Lymphoma

The histologic diagnosis of non-Hodgkin's lymphoma is difficult and requires an extensive sampling of lymphoid tissue with complicated immunohistochemical

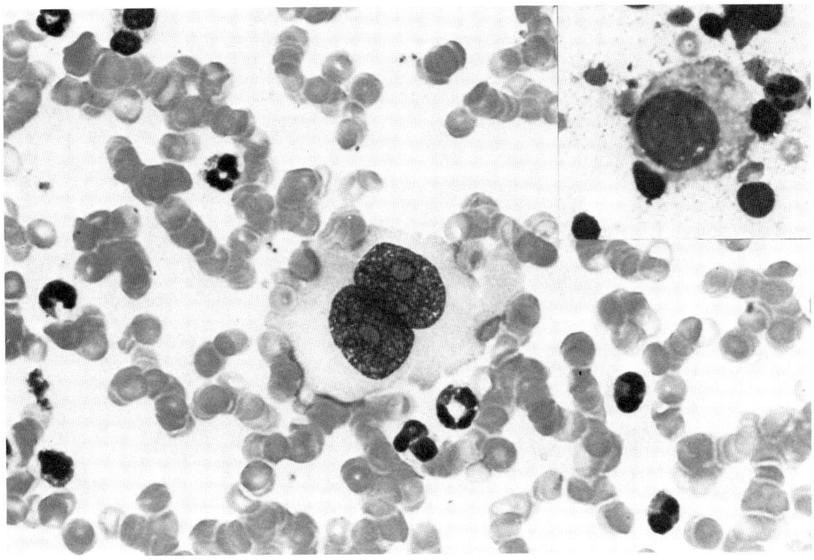

Figure 6-3. Hodgkin's disease. A Reed-Sternberg cell. **Inset:** a Hodgkin cell. (Giemsa ×500.)

studies. It is now widely accepted that NAB has limitations in the typing of non-Hodgkin's lymphoma.

In general, aspirate from a non-Hodgkin's lymphoma shows a monomorphic and dispersed malignant lymphoid cell population. However, there are cases in which making a cytologic distinction between a lymphoma and a florid reactive hyperplasia is very difficult or impossible. When a lymphoma cannot be ruled out with certainty by ABC, the affected lymph node must be excised for further studies. Among the several classifications of non-Hodgkin's lymphoma, the one proposed by Rappaport that does not identify the nodular or follicular pattern seen in histologic sections of the nodal tissue could be adapted for ABC.

A well-differentiated lymphoma yields tumor cells indistinguishable from normal lymphocytes. The only cytologic feature suggesting a lymphoma is the relative monomorphism of the aspirated lymphoid cells (Fig. 6-4). A poorly differentiated lymphoma will show large lymphoid cells with prominent nucleoli and mitoses (Fig. 6-5). Histiocytic or large cell lymphomas are readily identified by ABC. It reveals pleomorphic cells with vesicular nuclei showing irregular nuclear membranes, nuclear indentation, nuclear protrusion, coarsely clumped chromatin, and macronucleoli (Fig. 6-6).

Cytologic features of hyperplastic lymph node and lymphoma are summarized in Table 6-1.

METASTATIC CANCER

The cytodiagnosis of metastatic cancers in lymph nodes is usually straightforward by ABC. Identification of malignant cells as those that are not normally present in lymphoid tissue is relatively easy. Comparison of the cytologic or histologic

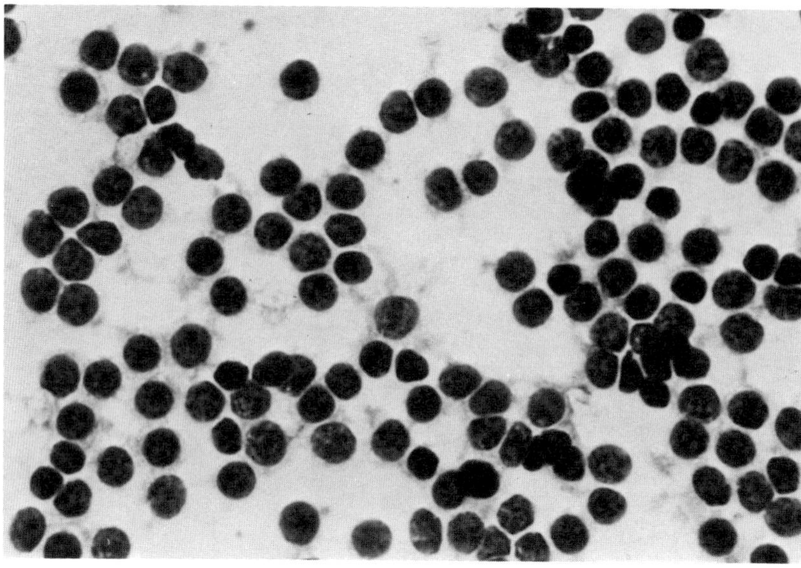

Figure 6-4. Well-differentiated non-Hodgkin's lymphoma. Monomorphic cell population consisting of small and benign-appearing lymphoid cells. (Papanicolaou ×500.)

material from the known primary tumor with the metastatic cancer cells aspirated from the affected lymph nodes usually leads to an accurate cytodiagnosis. Metastatic carcinoma of unknown primary is not an uncommon problem in clinical practice. In this situation the topography of the diseased lymph nodes and the types of metastatic cancer may be helpful in localizing the primary tumors. Metastases

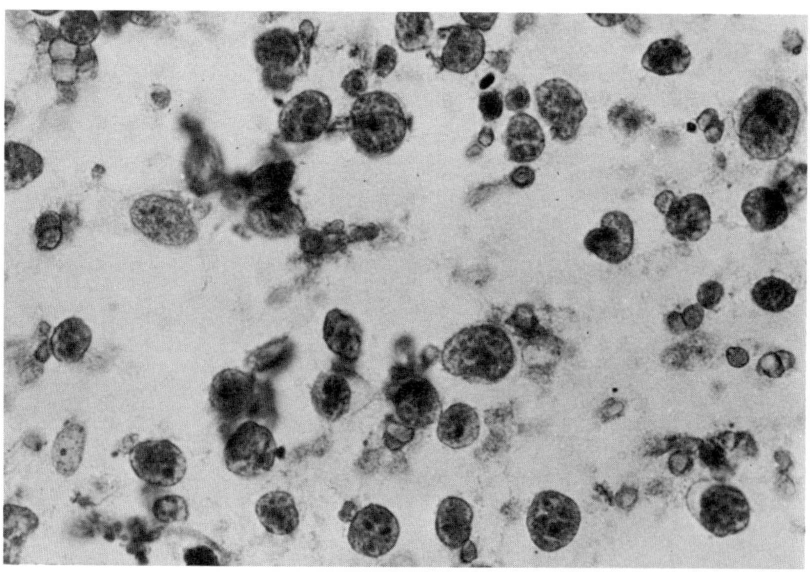

Figure 6-5. Poorly differentiated non-Hodgkin's lymphoma. Monomorphic cell population composed of malignant lymphoid cells showing nuclear irregularity and prominent nucleoli. (Papanicolaou ×500.)

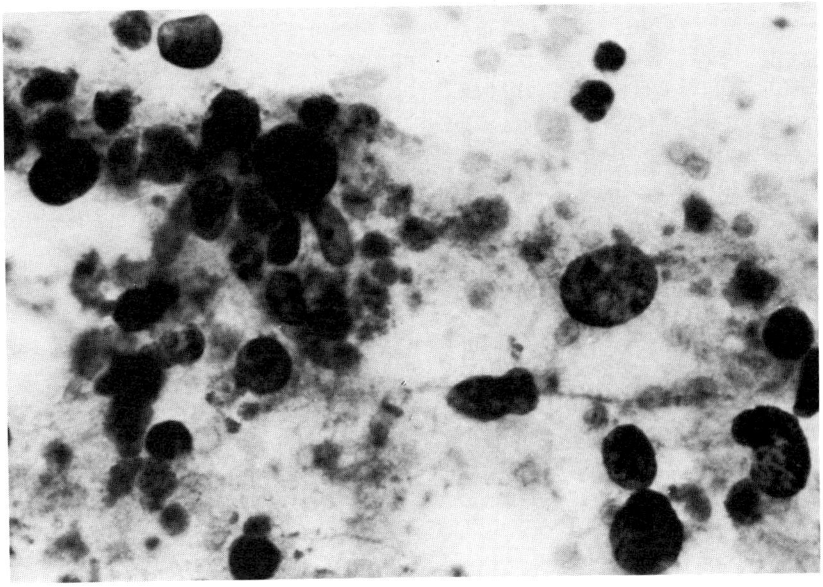

Figure 6-6. Large cell non-Hodgkin's lymphoma. Large malignant lymphoid cells. (Papanicolaou ×400.)

from glandular-type cancers of the kidney, thyroid, colon, and breast may display characteristic ABC findings, permitting a correct localization of the primary tumors in several cases. As a rule, most metastatic carcinomas in cervical lymph nodes in both adult males and females are associated with cancers of the oral cavity and upper respiratory tract, and most of them are squamous in type. Adenocarcinoma metastatic to cervical lymph nodes in men does not originate from any predominant site, while in women it commonly is associated with mammary carcinoma. The left supraclavicular lymph nodes are the common sites of metastatic gastrointestinal

Table 6-1. Comparative Cytomorphology of Hyperplastic Lymph Node and Lymphoma

ABC	HYPERPLASTIC LYMPH NODE	NON-HODGKIN'S LYMPHOMA	HODGKIN'S LYMPHOMA
Cells			
Population	Polymorphic	Monomorphic	Polymorphic
Characteristics	Lymphoid cells at variable development stages	Lymphoid cells	Lymphocytes Neutrophils Eosinophils Plasma cells
Special features	Macrophages with tingible bodies	Macronucleoli Nuclear indentation and protrusion	Reed-Sternberg cells Hodgkin cells

carcinomas. Metastatic carcinomas to lymph nodes below the clavicles are more commonly associated with cancers arising from the breast, lung, genital organs, gastrointestinal tract, and urinary tract. The mediastinum is the commonest site for metastatic lung cancers. However, carcinomas of other sites or organs may deposit in mediastinal lymph nodes. Retroperitoneal and pelvic lymph nodes are predominantly the sites for metastases of cancers arising from both male and female genitourinary systems. Inguinal lymph nodes drain mainly cancers of the external genitalia and anorectal region.

Squamous Cell Carcinoma

Well-differentiated and poorly differentiated carcinomas yield different ABC. Cells of a keratinizing well-differentiated carcinoma may present as single, large, and pleomorphic malignant squamous cells with orangeophilic cytoplasm (Fig. 6-7).

A poorly differentiated squamous carcinoma in contrast shows malignant epithelial cells in syncytia with ill-defined and nonkeratinizing cytoplasm (Fig. 6-8).

Adenocarcinoma

This type of tumor yields in NAB loose clusters of malignant cells showing ill-defined, vacuolated cytoplasm and enlarged nuclei with prominent nucleoli. The tumor cells may show papillary, acinar, or follicular groupings (Fig. 6-9). Metastatic breast carcinoma may display cells arranged in linear fashion and cells showing

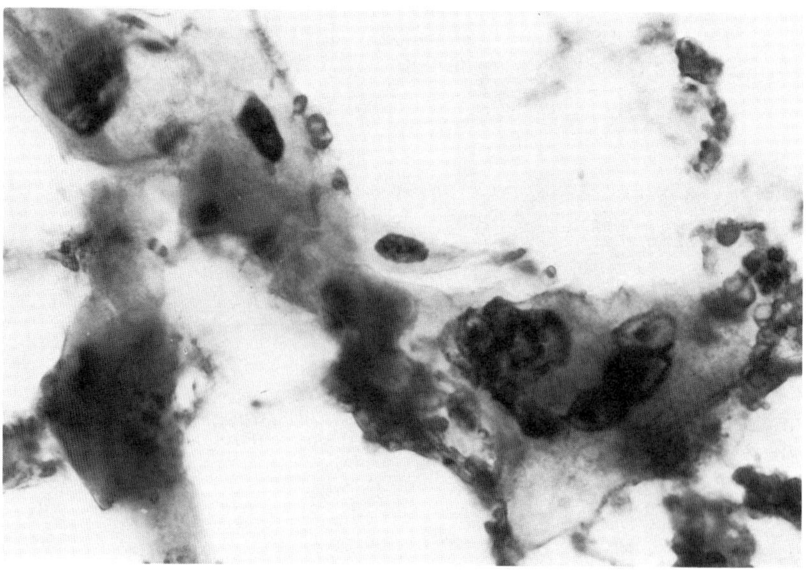

Figure 6-7. Metastatic well-differentiated squamous carcinoma to a cervical lymph node. Clustered keratinizing malignant squamous cells. (Papanicolaou ×400.)

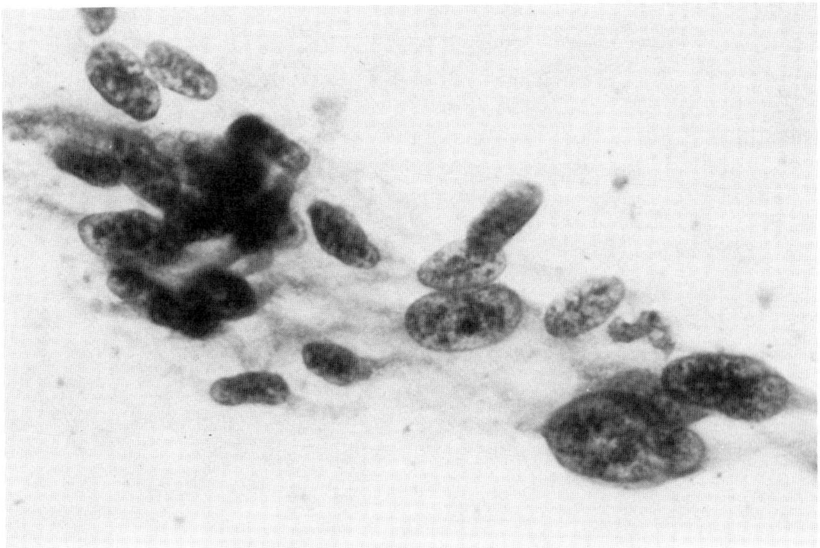

Figure 6-8. Metastatic poorly differentiated squamous carcinoma to a cervical lymph node. A syncytial group of malignant squamous cells with thin and ill-defined cytoplasm. (Papanicolaou ×400.)

intracytoplasmic vacuoles containing condensed mucous material. Cells of a renal cell carcinoma are seen in large monolayer sheets with vacuolated or clear cytoplasm (Fig. 6-10). Colonic adenocarcinoma commonly yields fragments of malignant glandular epithelium with columnar cells at the free borders arranged in palisade (Fig. 6-11).

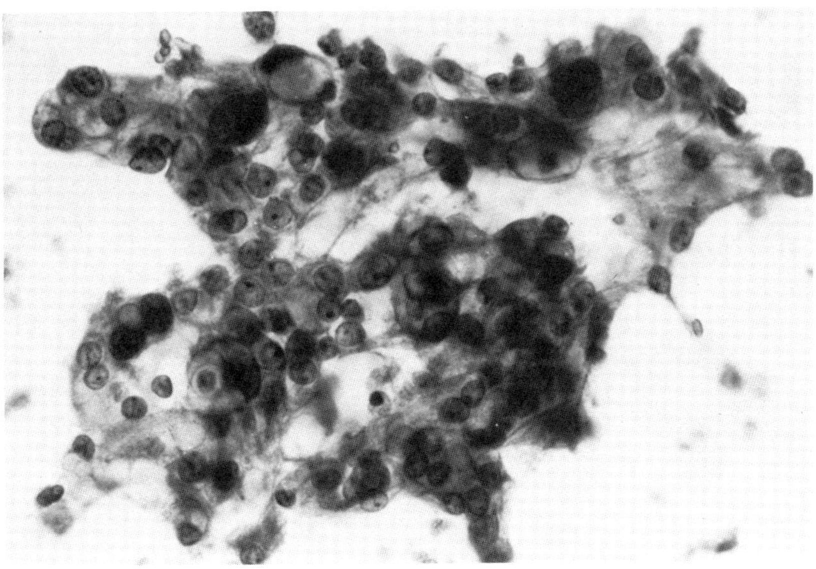

Figure 6-9. Metastatic bronchogenic adenocarcinoma to a supraclavicular lymph node. A large group of malignant glandular cells with focal acinar arrangement, cytoplasmic vacuoles, and nuclei with macronucleoli. (Papanicolaou ×250.)

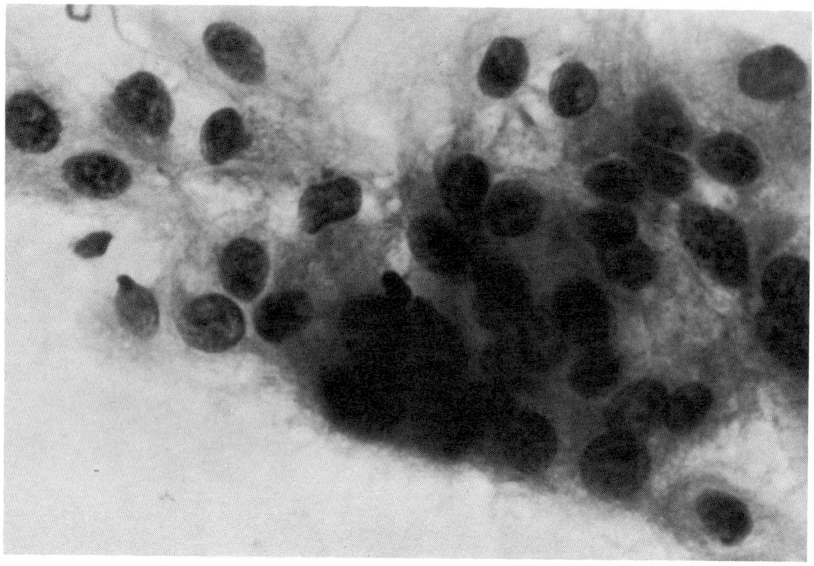

Figure 6-10. Metastatic renal cell carcinoma to a retroperitoneal lymph node. A large monolayered sheet of glandular-type cells showing clear, vacuolated or granular cytoplasm. (Papanicolaou ×400.)

Immunocytochemical study may be helpful in determining the site of the primary cancer sometimes. Cells of a metastatic prostatic adenocarcinoma and those of a metastatic thyroid carcinoma will stain positively with prostatic acid phosphatase or prostate-specific antigen, and thyroglobulin antisera, respectively. In a

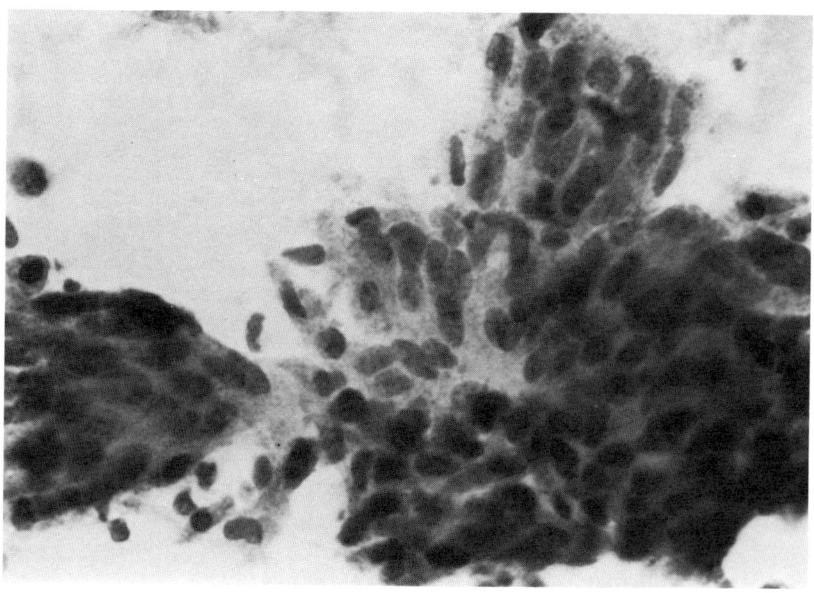

Figure 6-11. Metastatic colonic adenocarcinoma to a supraclavicular lymph node. A fragment of malignant glandular epithelium showing columnar cells at free borders arranged in palisade. (Papanicolaou ×250.)

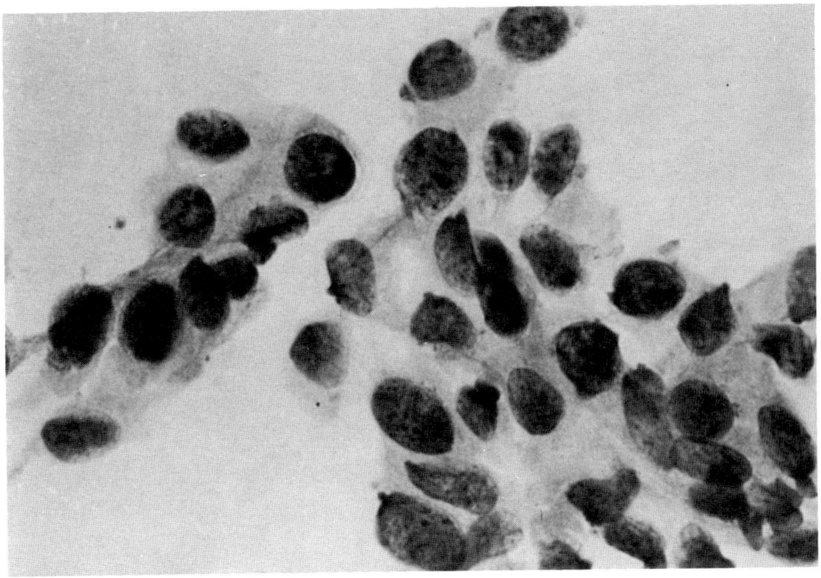

Figure 6-12. Metastatic transitional cell carcinoma grade 2 to a pelvic lymph node showing dyshesive sheets of malignant tumor cells. (Papanicolaou ×400.)

number of cases, however, the sites of the primary tumors cannot be suggested on the basis of ABC alone, and a full clinical investigation with radiologic imaging and pathological studies is necessary in these situations.

Transitional Cell Carcinoma

A transitional cell carcinoma grade 1 yields in NAB clusters of polygonal cells with well-defined abundant cytoplasm and vesicular nuclei displaying a finely granular chromatin pattern and inconspicuous nucleoli. Grade 2 tumors show loosely clustered and single malignant cells with well-defined cytoplasm and slightly pleomorphic nuclei (Fig. 6-12). Grade 3 tumors are characterized by pleomorphic malignant cells singly or in groups.

Anaplastic Carcinoma

Small and large cell anaplastic carcinomas commonly metastasize from the lung to hilar lymph nodes, sometimes from an occult primary focus. The NAB from lymph nodes harboring their metastases shows single and loosely clustered small or large cancer cells. Cellular molding and necrotic debris characterize the aspirate of the small cell tumor. Metastases from the large cell variety reveal considerably larger cells with scant cytoplasm and nuclei showing coarsely clumped chromatin and macronucleoli. Sometimes malignant multinucleated giant cells are seen (Fig. 6-13).

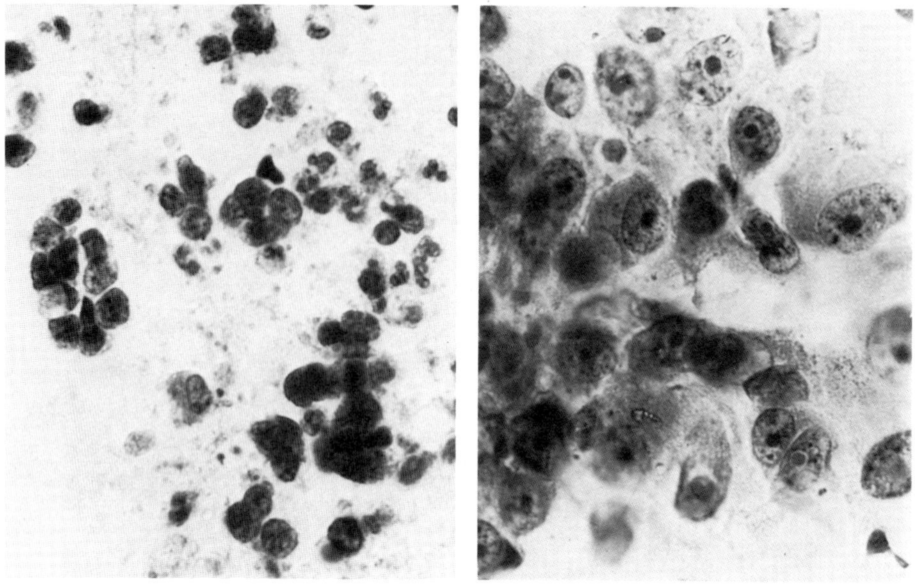

A B

Figure 6-13. Metastatic anaplastic bronchogenic carcinoma to cervical lymph nodes. **A.** Small cell tumor showing single and loosely clustered cells with nuclear molding and background debris. **B.** Large cell tumor showing cells with large nuclei and macronucleoli. (Papanicolaou ×400.)

Neuroendocrine Tumor

Neuroendocrine tumors can arise from different sites and encompass carcinoid tumors and oat cell carcinomas of the lung, gastrointestinal tract, genitourinary organs, and endocrine tumors of the pancreas, etc. The oat cell carcinoma is an aggressive neoplasm, and its ABC has just been discussed. The carcinoid tumor can be a slow-growing or aggressive tumor, depending on its origin: bronchogenic carcinoid tumors usually behave in a benign fashion while those of the gastrointestinal tract and pancreas are more aggressive. Aspirate from a metastatic neuroendocrine tumor of the stomach to a cervical lymph node reveals isolated and clustered monomorphic cells showing round nuclei and a moderate amount of cytoplasm that stains positively with neuron-specific enolase antiserum. Intracytoplasmic Grimelius-positive granules may also be demonstrated (Fig. 6-14).

Germ Cell Tumor

Germ cell tumors of the gonads commonly spread to pelvic and retroperitoneal lymph nodes. A seminoma or dysgerminoma shows in NAB single and clustered round and polygonal cells with round or vesicular nuclei with macronucleoli mixed with benign lymphoctyes (Fig. 6-15). An embryonal carcinoma of the testicle yields loose groups of malignant cells showing ill-defined cytoplasm and large nuclei with

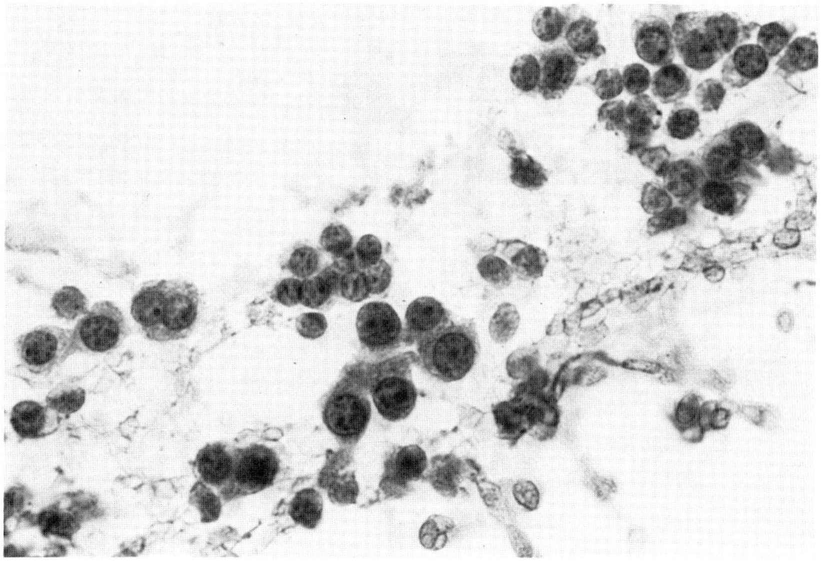

Figure 6-14. Metastatic neuroendocrine tumor of the stomach to a supraclavicular lymph node, showing isolated and clustered monomorphic neoplastic cells with round nuclei. (Papanicolaou ×400.)

macronucleoli (Fig. 6-16). A mature testicular teratoma displays in needle aspirate clusters of keratinized squames and groups of benign-appearing columnar glandular cells (Fig. 6-17). A choriocarcinoma may yield in NAB clusters of polygonal cytotrophoblastic cells and large multinucleated syncytiotrophoblastic cells (Fig. 6-18). The cytoplasm of embryonal carcinoma and choriocarcinoma cells almost

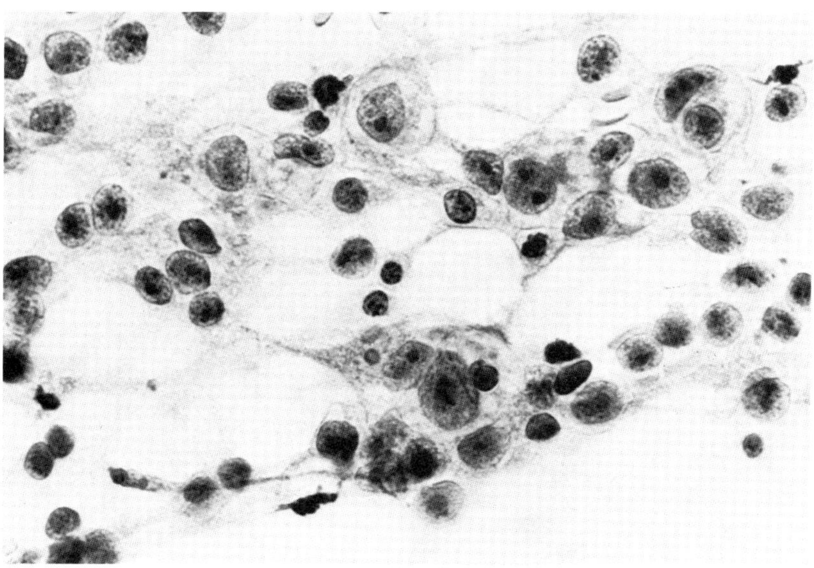

Figure 6-15. Metastatic seminoma to a retroperitoneal lymph node. Single and clustered polygonal tumor cells, showing macronucleoli. (Papanicolaou ×400.)

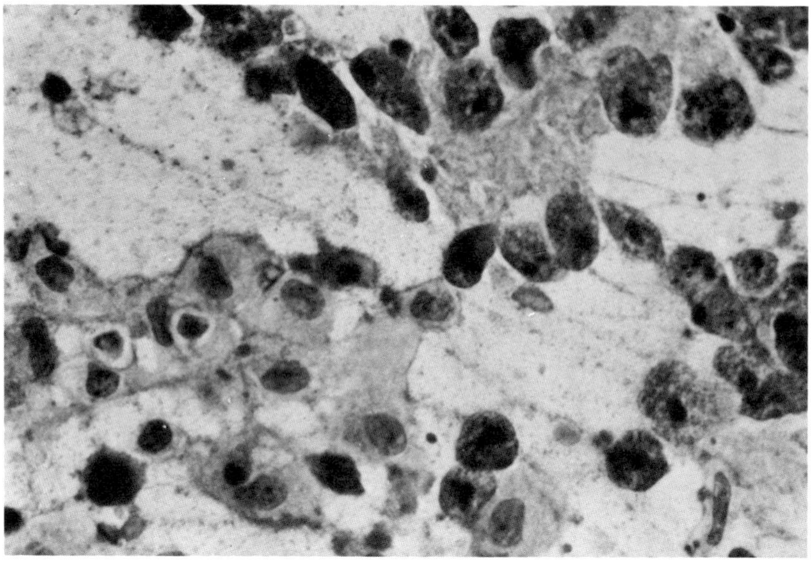

Figure 6-16. Metastatic embryonal carcinoma of the testis to a cervical lymph node. Loose group of tumor cells with ill-defined cytoplasm and pleomorphic nuclei. (Papanicolaou ×400.)

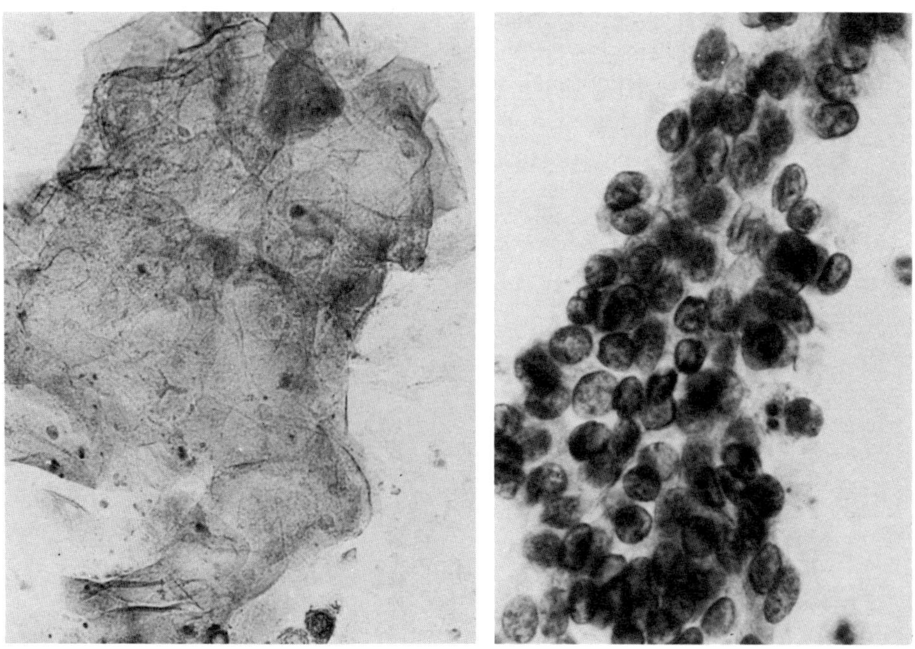

A B

Figure 6-17. Metastatic mature teratoma of the testis to a retroperitoneal lymph node. **A.** A cluster of anucleated squames. **B.** A fragment of bland but disordered glandular epithelium. (Papanicolaou ×250.)

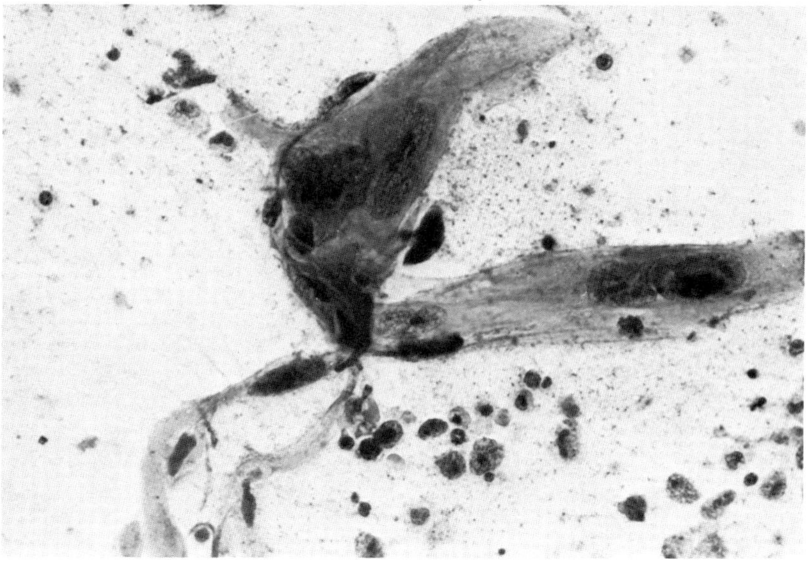

Figure 6-18. Metastatic testicular choriocarcinoma to a retroperitoneal lymph node. A group of syncytiotrophoblasts and a few isolated small cytotrophoblasts. (Papanicolaou ×250.)

always stains positively with β-HCG antiserum. An endodermal sinus tumor shows pleomorphic malignant cells singly and in clusters. Intracytoplasmic eosinophilic inclusions may be observed, and the tumor cell cytoplasm stains positively with α-fetoprotein antiserum.

Melanoma

Metastatic melanomas will yield abundant cellular material containing mainly isolated cells that may be oval, polygonal, or spindle-shaped, depending on the histologic types. Two or three distinct cell populations may be seen: small cells, resembling those of histiocytic lymphoma; moderate-sized cells, sometimes plasmacytoid in appearance; and giant cells. The tumor cells usually show large nuclei with macronucleoli. Binucleation and intranuclear cytoplasmic inclusions may be noted. Intracytoplasmic melanin pigment granules may be seen with routine Papanicolaou staining, and they are better visualized with Fontana stain. The tumor cell cytoplasm stains positively with S-100 protein antiserum (Fig. 6-19).

DIAGNOSTIC ACCURACY

The diagnostic accuracy of lymph node ABC depends largely on the quality and the adequacy of the aspirates. With good biopsy techniques the rate of unsatisfactory or inadequate NAB specimens is about 10% for palpable lymph nodes; these are most evident from the axilla, where deeply situated nodes easily slide away into

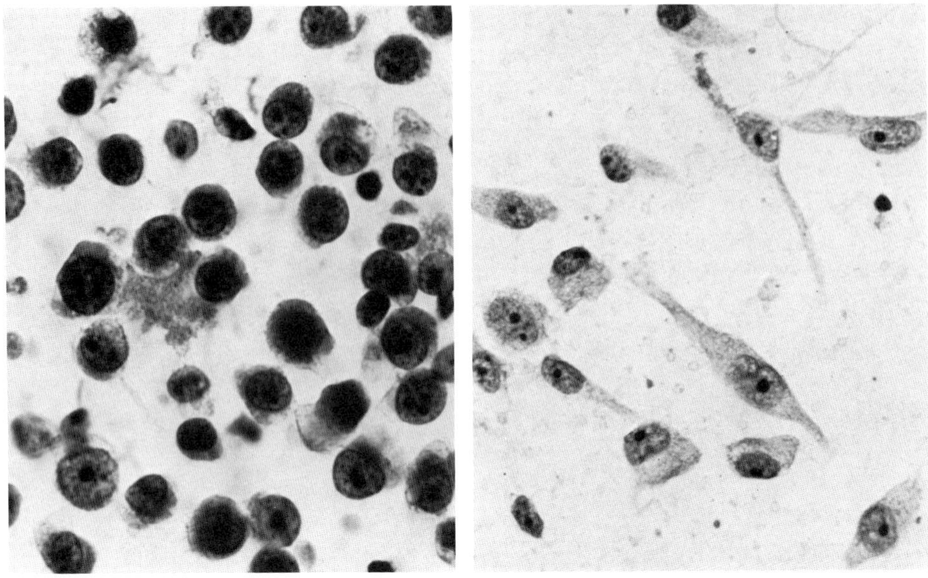

A B

Figure 6-19. Metastatic cutaneous malignant melanoma to regional lymph node. **A.** Isolated small oval tumor cells showing macronucleoli and one cell containing intracytoplasmic melanin pigment. **B.** Isolated, spindle-shaped, and plasmacytoid tumor cells with large nuclei and macronucleoli. (Papanicolaou ×400.)

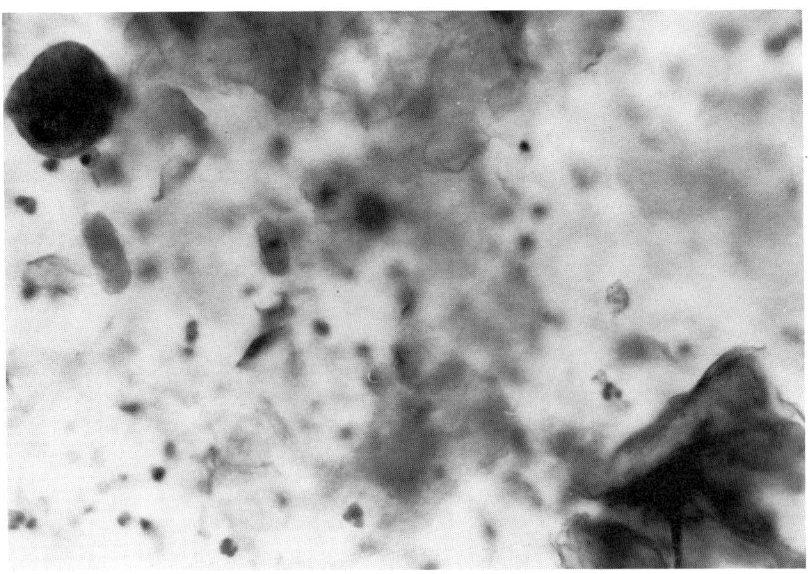

Figure 6-20. Ruptured epidermal inclusion cyst with granulomatous reaction to keratinous material, showing keratinized squames and a multinucleated macrophage. (Papanicolaou ×400.)

the surrounding fat. For intrathoracic, retroperitoneal, and pelvic lymph nodes the rate of unsatisfactory aspiration specimens is higher because of the difficulty of sampling technique, and it is also related to the experience of the aspirator.

In experienced hands, the sensitivity of NAB in the diagnosis of Hodgkin's disease can reach 80%, especially in lymphocytic depletion and mixed cellularity variants. For non-Hodgkin's lymphoma the diagnostic accuracy varies with the degree of the tumor differentiation: up to 36% of well-differentiated lymphomas mimic reactive hyperplasia, while 90% of large-cell or histiocytic lymphomas can be identified by ABC. Metastatic cancers to lymph nodes are relatively easily identified by NAB. The diagnostic accuracy may reach 99% with adequate specimens.

DIAGNOSTIC PITFALLS

False-negative results are about 5% in cases of malignant disease involving superficial lymph nodes and result from lack of experience, sampling errors, and fibrosis. Some cases of well-differentiated squamous carcinoma yield cells that may be mistaken for those of benign lesions, such as an epidermal inclusion cyst (Fig. 6-20) or a branchial cleft cyst. The presence of a cell-rich monomorphic population and a few pleomorphic anucleated "ghost" keratinized cells and erratically shaped cells with hyperchromatic bizarre nuclei will point to a squamous cancer (Fig. 6-21). A metastatic poorly differentiated squamous cancer may undergo extensive necrosis and shows in NAB numerous inflammatory cells and naked tumor cell nuclei. The presence of a few bizarre keratinizing cells is indicative of a metastatic squamous cell carcinoma (Fig. 6-22).

False-positive diagnoses are rare and may occur as the result of inexperience and unusual presentations of a benign process. Hyperplastic lymphoid tissue may yield monomorphic lymphocytes readily mistaken for those of a well-differentiated non-Hodgkin's lymphoma. Histiocytes and immature lymphoid cells from germinal centers of a toxoplasmic lymphadenitis may mimic cell composition of a malignant lymphoma. Aspirate from enlarged lymph nodes of patients with infectious mononucleosis or tuberculous lymphadenitis may show atypical histiocytes, simulating Reed-Sternberg cells. When the diagnosis of a benign lymphoid lesion is in doubt, excisional biopsy of the affected lymph node must be done for histologic confirmation.

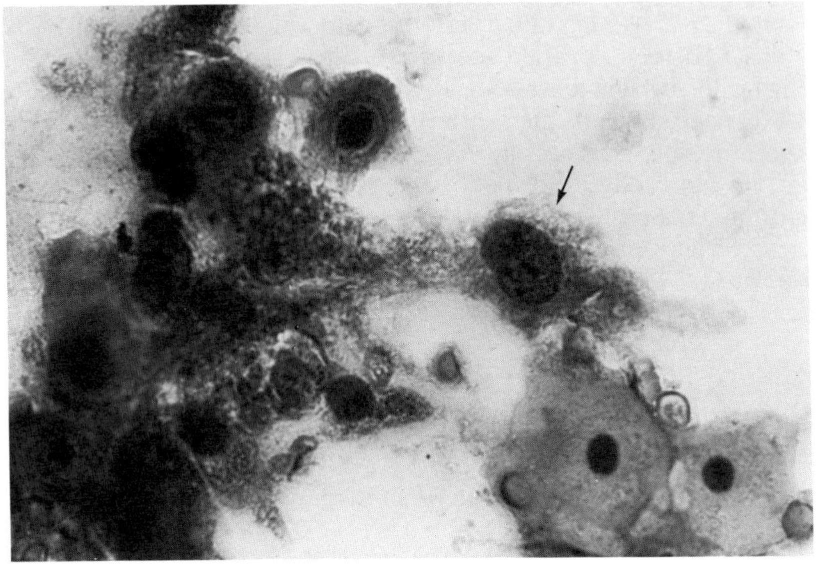

Figure 6-21. Metastatic well-differentiated squamous cell carcinoma of the oral cavity to a cervical lymph node, showing numerous benign-appearing polygonal squamous cells and a few bizarre malignant cells (*arrow*). (Papanicolaou ×400.)

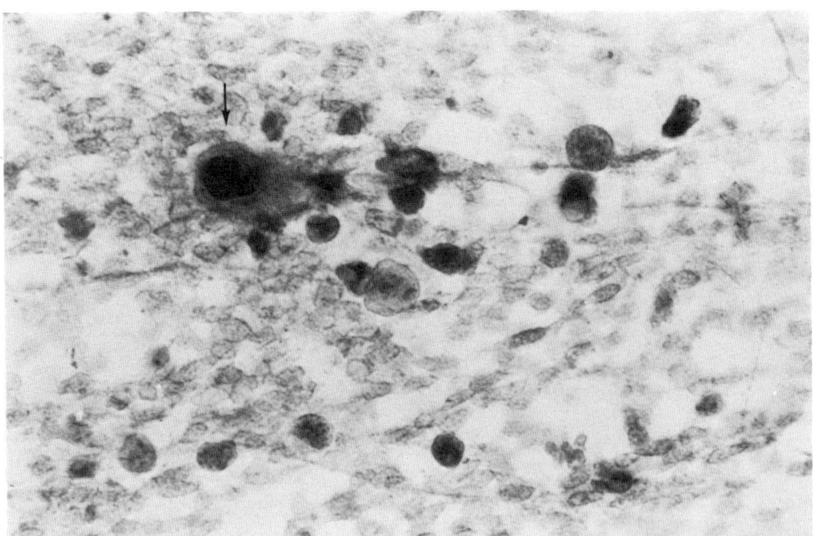

Figure 6-22. Metastatic poorly differentiated squamous cell carcinoma to a cervical lymph node with extensive necrosis. Note several naked nuclei and a malignant keratinizing squamous cell (*arrow*). (Papanicolaou ×400.)

SUGGESTED READING

Betsill WL, Hajdu SI: Percutaneous aspiration biopsy of lymph nodes. *Am J Clin Pathol* 1980;73:471–479.

Bonfiglio TA, Dvoretsky PM, Piscioli F, et al.: Fine needle aspiration biopsy in the evaluation of lymphoreticular tumors of the thorax. *Acta Cytol* 1985;29:548–553.

Bonfiglio TA, MacIntosh PK, Patten SF Jr, et al.: Fine needle aspiration cytopathology of retroperitoneal lymph nodes in the evaluation of metastatic disease. *Acta Cytol* 1979;23:126–130.

Engzell U, Jakobsson PA, Sigurdson A, et al.: Aspiration biopsy of metastatic carcinoma in lymph nodes of the neck. A review of 1101 consecutive cases. *Acta Otolaryngol* 1981;72:138–147.

Friedman M, Kim U, Shimaoka K, et al.: Appraisal of aspiration cytology in management of Hodgkin's disease. *Cancer* 1980;45:1653–1663.

Kline TS, Kannan V: Aspiration biopsy cytology of melanoma. *Am J Clin Pathol* 1982;77:597–601.

Kline TS, Kannan V, Kline IK: Lymphadenopathy and aspiration biopsy cytology: review of 376 superficial nodes. *Cancer* 1984;54:1076–1081.

Kline TS: *Handbook of Fine Needle Aspiration Biopsy Cytology*, ed 2. New York, Churchill Livingstone, 1988, pp 49–120.

Nguyen GK: Fine needle aspiration biopsy cytology of metastatic renal cell carcinoma. *Acta Cytol* 1988;32:409–414.

Qizilbash AH, Elavathil LJ, Chen V, et al.: Aspiration biopsy cytology of lymph nodes in malignant lymphoma. *Diagn Cytopathol* 1985;1:18–22.

Ramzy I, Rove R, Schultenover SJ, et al.: Lymph node aspiration biopsy. Diagnostic reliability and limitations. *Diagn Cytopathol* 1985;1:39–45.

Suen KC: *Guides to Clinical Aspiration Biopsy: Retroperitoneum and Intestine*. New York, Igaku-Shoin, 1987, pp 23–100.

7

BONE AND SOFT TISSUE

In this chapter the cytologic aspects of bone and soft tissue tumors will be discussed together because many primary sarcomas of soft tissue are also found in bone. The role of NAB in confirming a metastatic carcinoma to bones is widely accepted. However, its value in the correct typing of primary tumors of bone and soft tissue suffers severe limitations. These neoplasms often display complicated histologic patterns, and their final diagnoses require an extensive tissue sampling with immunohistochemical and electron microscopic studies, as well as a close roentgenographic correlation. Although tumors of bone and soft tissue are numerous, only a few commonly encountered in clinical practice are hereby discussed and illustrated.

BONE

Indications for NAB

NAB is used for morphologic confirmation of a clinically and roentgenologically malignant primary or metastatic bone tumor prior to institution of an appropriate treatment. It may be used to confirm the benign nature of a radiologically benign bone neoplasm. If the tumor undergoing biopsy is not clearly identified by ABC, however, tissue biopsy must be performed for definite diagnosis.

Primary Bone Tumors

Osteogenic sarcoma. The tumor usually occurs at the metaphysis of long bones in young adults. It may develop in bones with prior radiation and in older patients who have Paget's bone disease. It usually has a characteristic roentgenography. Histologically, it is composed of different types of cancer cells producing osteoid and bone. NAB reveals necrotic debris, numerous blood cells, and usually several pleomorphic, epithelioid, chondroblastic, or small nonepithelial malignant cells present singly, in loose or tight clusters (Fig. 7-1A and B). Osteoid is rarely identifiable with confidence. Therefore, an accurate diagnosis of osteogenic sarcoma cannot be made on ABC alone.

Giant cell tumor. This tumor with both benign and malignant variants usually occurs at the epiphysis of long bones in patients over 20 years old and has special roentgenographic characteristics. The aspirate reveals numerous large, osteoclast-type, multinucleated giant cells and spindle-shaped stromal cells that are present singly and in clusters (Fig. 7-2A and B). Depending on the cytologic features of the stromal cells the neoplasm may be classified as benign or malignant. It is important to remember that the presence of multinucleated giant cells is a fairly nonspecific finding, because these cells may be seen in many benign and malignant bone lesions. Clinical data and roentgenologic features of bone tumors must be taken into consideration when their ABC is evaluated.

Chondrosarcoma. This tumor is more commonly found in the pelvic bone, humerus, and ribs. Occasionally, it arises from a preexisting osteochondroma. Its ABC varies with the degree of tumor differentiation. A well-differentiated chondrosarcoma yields cells mimicking benign chondrocytes and may not be distinguishable from a chondroma. Cells aspirated from a poorly differentiated tumor are readily identifiable as malignant cartilaginous cells with well-defined vacuolated cytoplasm and single or multiple bizarre nuclei containing macronucleoli. They may have a signet-ring configuration resembling cells of an anaplastic gastric carcinoma; mucicarmine stain, however, is negative (Fig. 7-3A).

Chordoma. This tumor of notochordal origin is more common in men over 30 years of age. Its most frequent location is the sacrococcygeal region, followed by the skull base and cervical vertebrae. Sacrococcygeal chordomas often have a presacral extension, and they can be sampled by transrectal NAB. Aspirated material is gelatinous and shows numerous physaliferous cells with large intracytoplasmic vacuoles pushing the nuclei to the periphery of the cells. The nuclei are pleomorphic, single, or multiple with or without macronucleoli (Fig. 7-3B). The cells should be distinguished from those of a mucus-secreting adenocarcinoma and chondrosarcoma; the mucicarmine stain can be helpful.

Ewing's sarcoma. This neoplasm occurs mainly in tubular long bones of children and adolescents and displays characteristic roentgenologic features. NAB from the tumor shows small round cells dispersed or arranged in clusters or in a rosette-like pattern. The individual tumor cell is 2 to 3 times larger than a mature lymphocyte. The relatively scant cytoplasm is periodic acid-Schiff positive. Differential diagnosis should include neuroblastoma and lymphoma (Fig. 7-4A).

Multiple myeloma. This disease occurs in patients over 40 years of age and usually affects ribs, vertebral column, skull, and pelvic bone. It produces multiple punch-out osteolytic lesions. About 90% of patients have multiple lesions and dysproteinemia with a M spike on serum protein electrophoresis. NAB from the lesion detects numerous dispersed atypical or bizarre plasma cells (Fig. 7-4B).

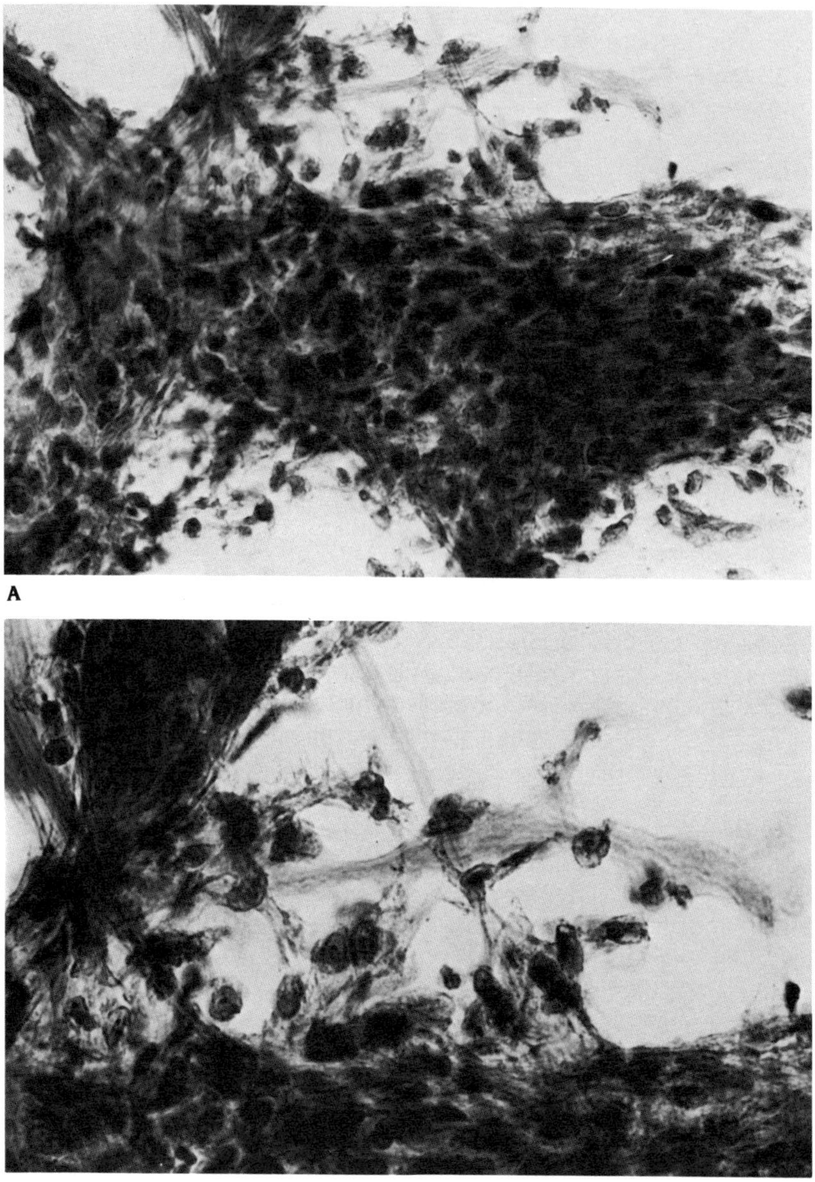

A

B

Figure 7-1. Osteogenic sarcoma. **A.** An irregular cluster of malignant fibroblast-like cells. **B.** Higher magnification of the same cell group, showing cellular pleomorphism (Papanicolaou: **A.** ×250. **B.** ×400.)

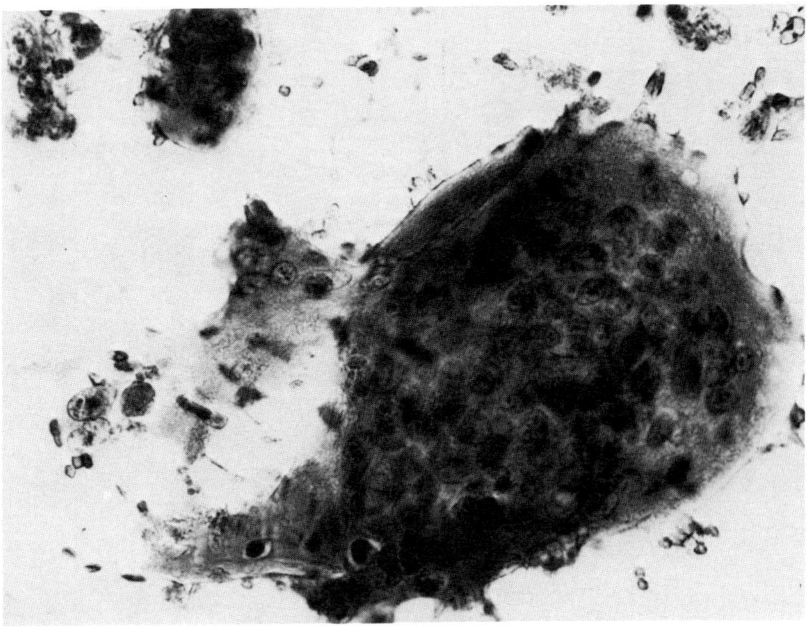

A

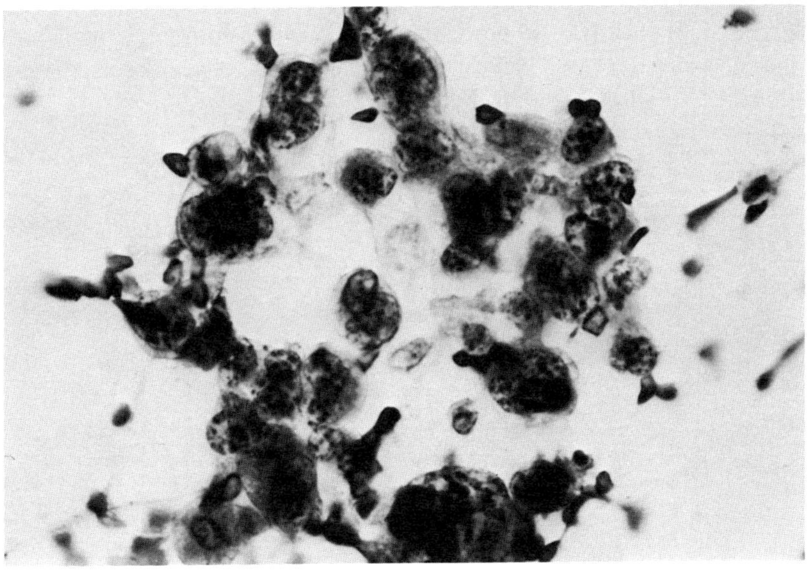

B

Figure 7-2. Malignant giant cell tumor of bone. **A.** Large multinucleated giant cells. **B.** Pleomorphic malignant stromal cells. (Papanicolaou: **A.** ×250. **B.** ×400.)

Metastatic Cancers

Metastatic cancers to bone may be readily confirmed by NAB. Carcinomas of breast, prostate, lung, kidney, and thyroid may metastasize to bones. These metastases can occur in any bones, and about 70% of them affect the axial skeleton

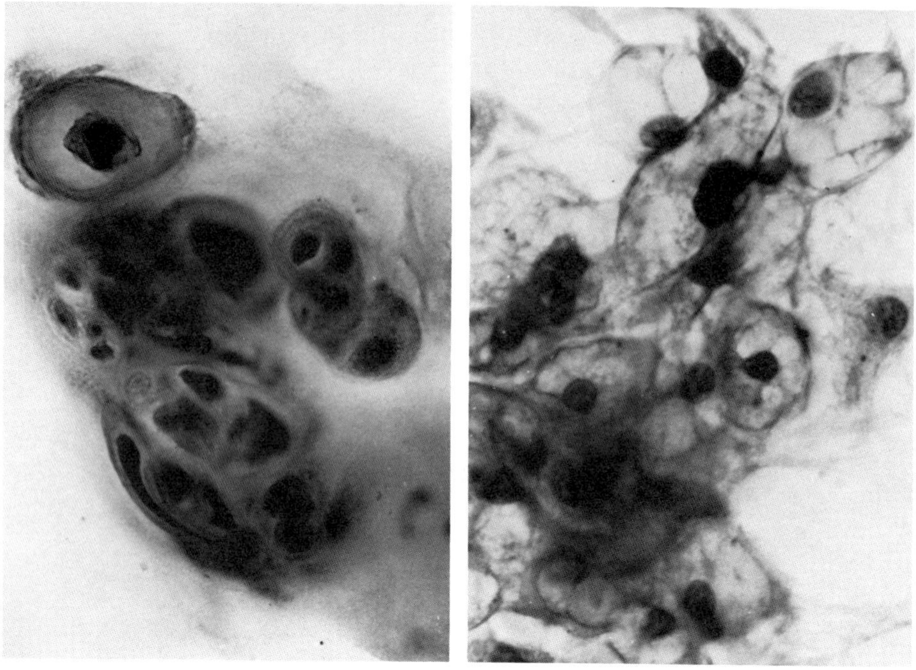

A B

Figure 7-3. **A.** High-grade chondrosarcoma showing pleomorphic malignant cartilaginous cells. **B.** Chordoma showing characteristic physaliferous tumor cells. (Papanicolaou: **A.** ×250. **B.** ×400.)

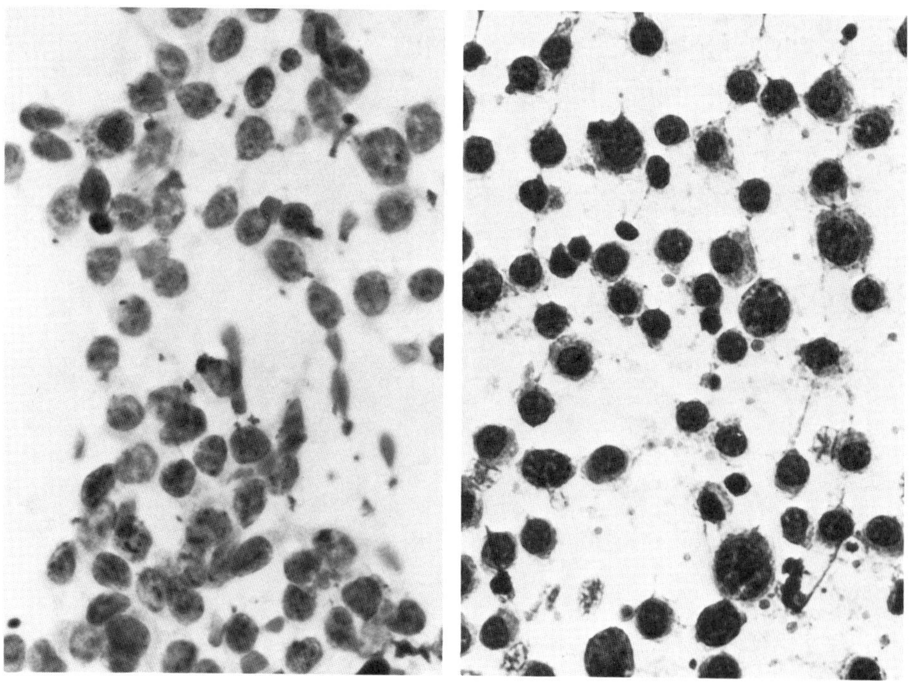

A B

Figure 7-4. **A.** Ewing's sarcoma showing dispersed round tumor cells. **B.** Multiple myeloma displaying single pleomorphic plasma cells. (**A.** Papanicolaou ×400. **B.** Hematoxylin and eosin, ×400.)

(cranium, ribs, spine, and sacrum). They are more commonly seen as multiple osteolytic lesions and, rarely, as osteoblastic lesions. However, solitary metastases from occult primaries can simulate primary bone cancers. The ABC of those metastatic cancers is similar to that of tumors of the same histologic types (see Chapter 6, Metastatic Cancer).

Diagnostic Accuracy and Pitfalls

The cytodiagnostic accuracy of bone tumors (benign vs. malignant) is about 80% in experienced hands. It is as high as that of trephine biopsy. Special diagnostic problems of bone tumors have just been discussed individually.

SOFT TISSUE

Indications for NAB

In general, NAB of soft tissue neoplasms has limited value in accurate tumor typing. Often, however, it assists in clinical management, and for lipomatous tumors, a correct diagnosis by ABC is possible in a large number of cases. ABC usually can discriminate a benign from a malignant tumor, and it is possible to classify soft tissue sarcomas in broad categories of pleomorphic, spindle-cell, and round-cell types. This rather simple classification is important to the oncologist because it has been demonstrated that, regardless of the histogenesis, soft tissue sarcomas with certain predominant cell types tend to respond to some classes of chemotherapeutic agents and/or radiation therapy. For example, round-cell sarcomas of childhood respond well to a combined irradiation with an alkylating agent, whereas spindle-cell sarcomas are resistant to radiation and chemotherapy. When the tumor studied is classified into one of these three main groups, appropriate cytochemical and immunocytochemical studies and electron microscopic examination of aspirated tumor cells may be helpful to further confirm the suspected cytodiagnosis.

NAB is not critical in the diagnosis and management of superficial soft tissue tumors, as they can be easily excised under local anesthesia. Deeply located mass lesions in the abdominal cavity, retroperitoneum, and limbs, however, may be well-assessed by NAB. An inflammatory mass, for example, can be correctly diagnosed by ABC and is appropriately treated with antibiotics.

Lipomatous Tumors

The majority of deeply located and retroperitoneal lipomatous neoplasms are malignant. Usually, with representative cell samples a lipoma and a liposarcoma can be diagnosed with confidence.

Lipoma yields in NAB irregular large clusters of benign fat cells with small eccentrically located, regular nuclei.

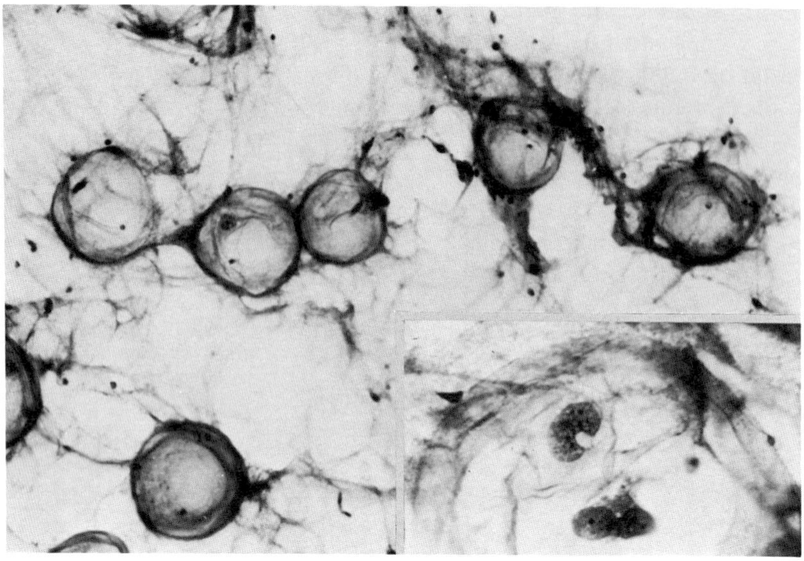

Figure 7-5. Well-differentiated liposarcoma showing isolated fat cells with enlarged nuclei. **Inset:** High magnification of two tumor cells, one showing two nuclei. (Papanicolaou ×100, **Inset** ×400.)

Liposarcomas have four main subtypes: Well-differentiated, myxomatous, round-cell, and pleomorphic. These histologic variants display different cytologic patterns in ABC. Well-differentiated tumors are characterized by several groups of fat cells showing enlarged, slightly pleomorphic, hyperchromatic, and mono- or bilobed nuclei. Naked, irregular, hyperchromatic nuclei, and anastomotic capillary

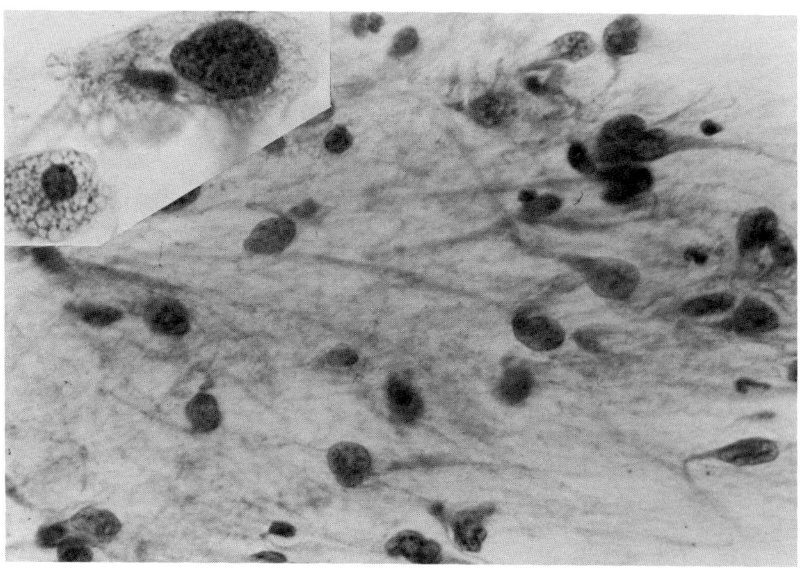

Figure 7-6. Myxomatous liposarcoma showing small round tumor cells in myxomatous background. **Inset:** lipoblasts. (Papanicolaou ×400.)

blood vessels are also noted (Fig. 7-5). A myxomatous tumor shows abundant myxomatous material containing round or bizarre-appearing lipoblasts with enlarged, hyperchromatic, irregular nuclei, and vacuolated cytoplasm and anastomosing capillary blood vessels (Fig. 7-6). NAB from a round-cell tumor reveals mainly small cancer cells with scant cytoplasm. A careful examination will detect vacuolated lipoblasts. Pleomorphic liposarcoma as indicated by its name shows in NAB pleomorphic cancer cells, with many of them containing intracytoplasmic fat vacuoles. An oil red-O staining of air-dried smears is very helpful in making a correct diagnosis of lipomatous tumors.

Spindle-Cell Tumors

Fibroblastic and smooth-muscle cell tumors yield in NAB single and clustered spindle-shaped cells.

Cells of *fibroma* and *fibrosarcoma* are characterized by their spindle-shaped nuclei, displaying benign and malignant nuclear features, respectively (Fig. 7-7).

Leiomyoma and low-grade *leiomyosarcoma* show single and clustered cells with cigar-shaped or blunt-ended nuclei. Malignant or bizarre nuclei are seen in NAB of the latter (Fig. 7-8).

Benign and malignant *nerve sheath tumors* show spindle cells present singly or in tissue fragments. In some cases the tumor cell nuclei are seen arranged in palisade. Nuclear pleomorphism is observed in both malignant and long-standing or ancient neurilemomas (Fig. 7-9). It constitutes a diagnostic pitfall in some cases of highly cellular ancient neurilemoma.

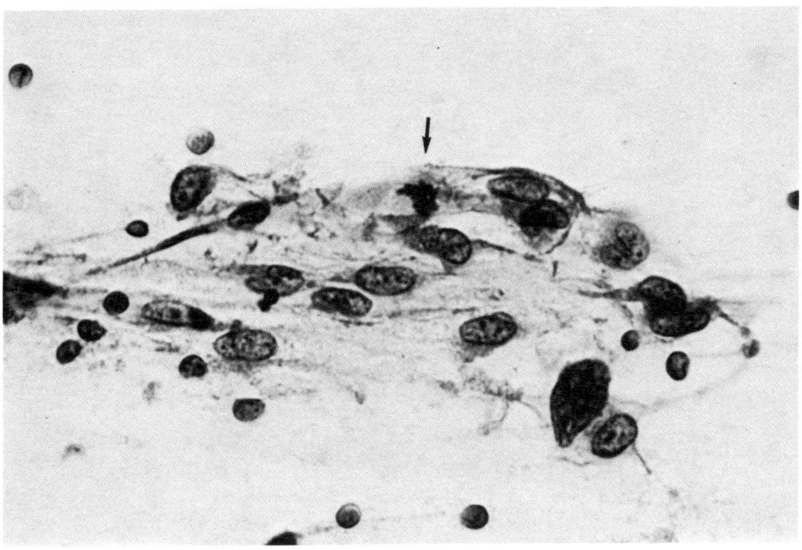

Figure 7-7. Fibrosarcoma showing single and loosely clustered tumor cells with elongated or spindle-shaped nuclei. A mitosis is present (*arrow*) (Papanicolaou ×400).

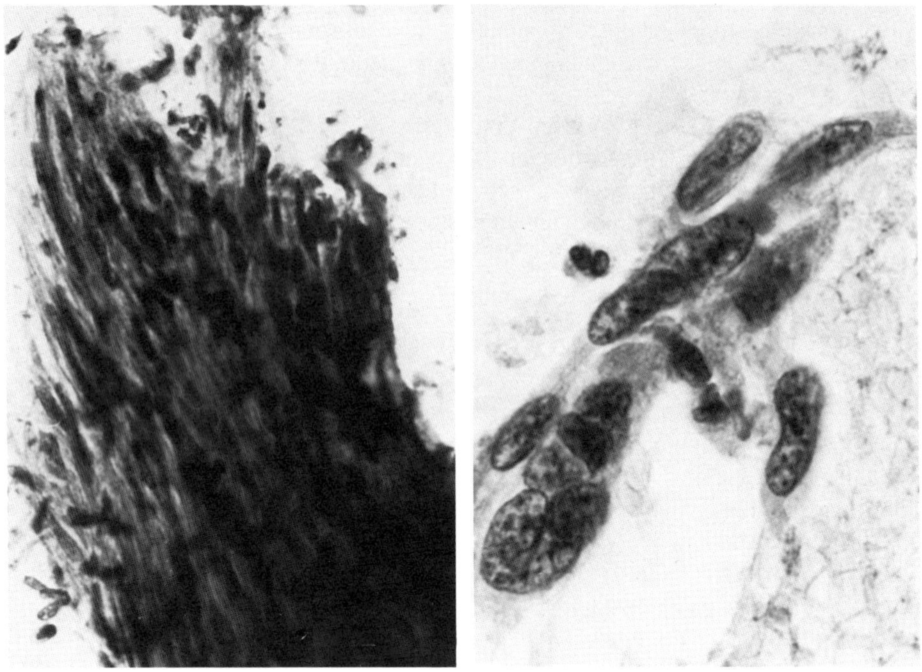

A B

Figure 7-8. **A.** Leiomyoma shows a group of benign smooth muscle cells with cigar-shaped nuclei. **B.** Leiomyosarcoma displays a cluster of elongated malignant tumor cells. (Papanicolaou: **A.** ×250. **B.** ×400.)

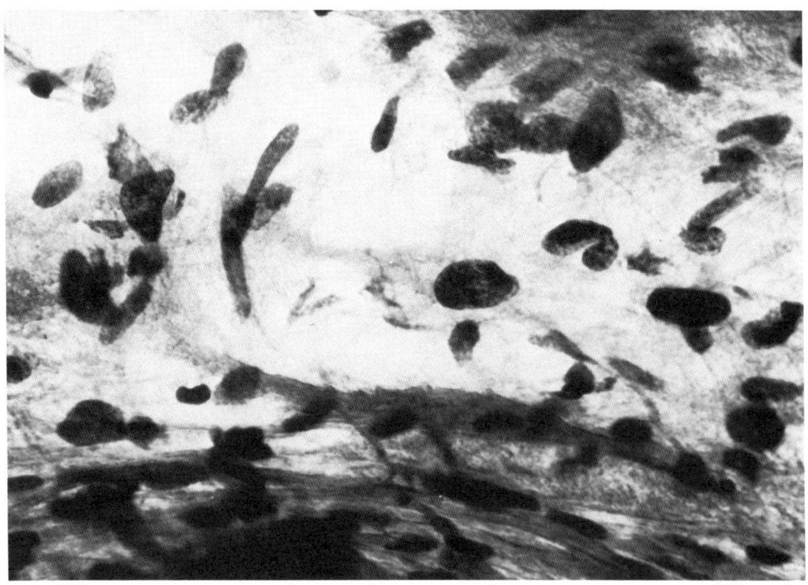

Figure 7-9. Ancient neurilemoma showing single and clustered elongated cells with ill-defined cytoplasm and pleomorphic hyperchromatic nuclei. (Hematoxylin and eosin, ×400.)

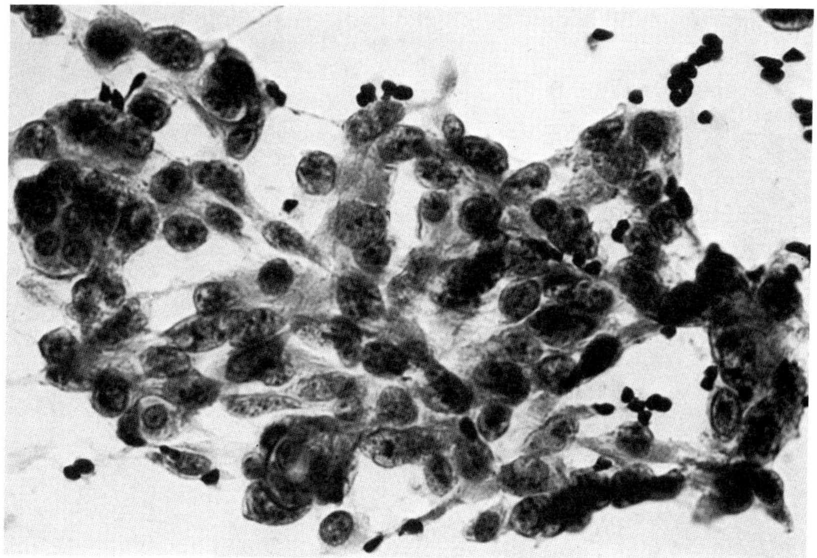

Figure 7-10. Angiosarcoma showing spindle-shaped malignant cells singly and in clusters. (Papanicolaou ×400.)

Angioma and *angiosarcoma* usually yield in NAB single or clustered spindle-shaped cells. However, pleomorphic and polygonal cells may be seen in ABC of the latter tumor. They may stain positively with factor VIII and lectin antisera (Fig. 7-10).

The cytodiagnosis of spindle-cell tumors is difficult with routinely stained smears. Cytochemical, immunocytochemical, and electron microscopic studies are helpful in tumor typing. Cytologic and ultrastructural characteristics of some commonly encountered spindle-cell tumors are summarized in Table 7-1.

Pleomorphic Tumors

Benign fibrous histiocytomas are usually located in the subcutaneous tissue. *Malignant fibrohistiocytomas* are usually deeply located in large muscle masses of the limbs and retroperitoneum and have three histologic variants: fibromatous, myxoid, and giant-cell. ABC shows little difference in terms of cellular composition. Basically, malignant fibroblast-like and histiocyte-like cells are seen in different proportions. The number of multinucleated giant tumor cells is variable, being abundant in the giant-cell type (Fig. 7-11).

Synovial sarcoma is a biphasic tumor, and its ABC is characterized in typical cases by single and clustered spindle-shaped cells with vesicular nuclei and macronucleoli and by sheets of polygonal glandular-type cells showing nuclei fairly similar to those of the spindle-shaped cells (Fig. 7-12A and B).

Other pleomorphic tumors consist of pleomorphic rhabdomyosarcoma, high-grade leiomyosarcoma, clear-cell sarcoma of soft parts, and epithelioid sarcoma. Cytologic features, including cytochemical, immunocytochemical, and electron microscopic features, of some common pleomorphic sarcomas are shown in Table 7-2.

Table 7-1. Cytologic Differential Diagnosis of Spindle-Cell Tumors

TUMOR	ABC	CYTOCHEMICAL AND IMMUNOCYTOCHEMICAL FEATURES	ELECTRON MICROSCOPIC FEATURES
Fibroma and fibrosarcoma	Single and clustered cells Spindled nuclei	Vimentin, +	Abundant rough endoplasmic reticula Indented, convoluted nuclei
Leiomyoma and leiomyosarcoma	Single and clustered cells Blunt-ended nuclei	Smooth muscle myosin, + Desmin, +	Bundles of microfilaments with focal densities
Neurogenic tumors	Single cells Tissue fragments Elongated, palisaded nuclei	S-100 protein, + Myelin basic protein, + Laminin, +	Elongated cytoplasmic processes with redundant basal laminae
Spindle-cell melanoma	Single cells Melanin Nuclear cytoplasmic inclusions Macronucleoli	Fontana, + intracytoplasmic granules S-100 protein, +	Melanosomes and premelanosomes
Angioma and angiosarcoma	Single and clustered cells	Factor VIII-related antigen, + *Ulex europaeus* agglutinin 1, +	Rod-shaped tubular bodies

Round-Cell Tumors

Extraskeletal Ewing's sarcoma, embryonal rhabdomyosarcoma, neuroblastoma, round cell liposarcoma, and soft-tissue non-Hodgkin's lymphoma are the main neoplasms of this group.

NAB from an *extraskeletal Ewing's sarcoma* reveals cells similar to those of a skeletal Ewing's tumor (Fig. 7-4A). An embryonal rhabdomyosarcoma shows single cells with fairly abundant and eosinophilic cytoplasm. N*euroblastoma* is characterized

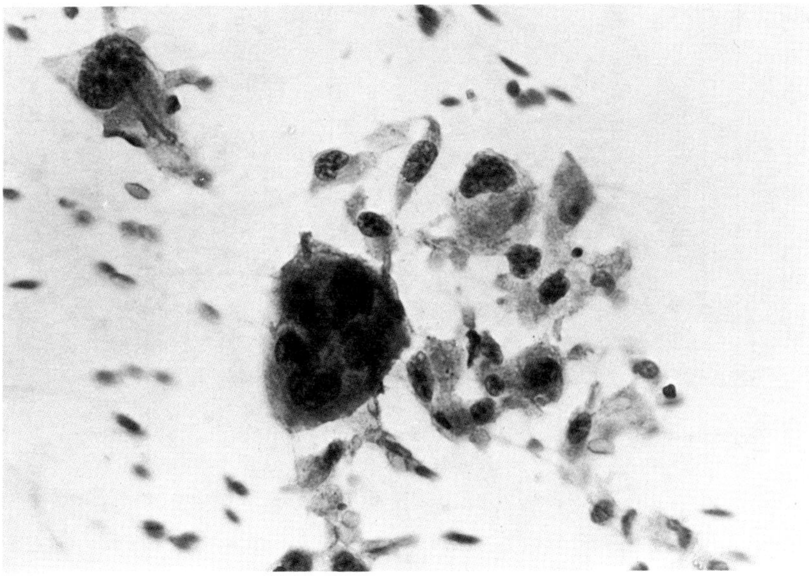

Figure 7-11. Malignant fibrous histiocytoma showing a pleomorphic cell population with a large multinucleated giant cell. (Papanicolaou ×400.)

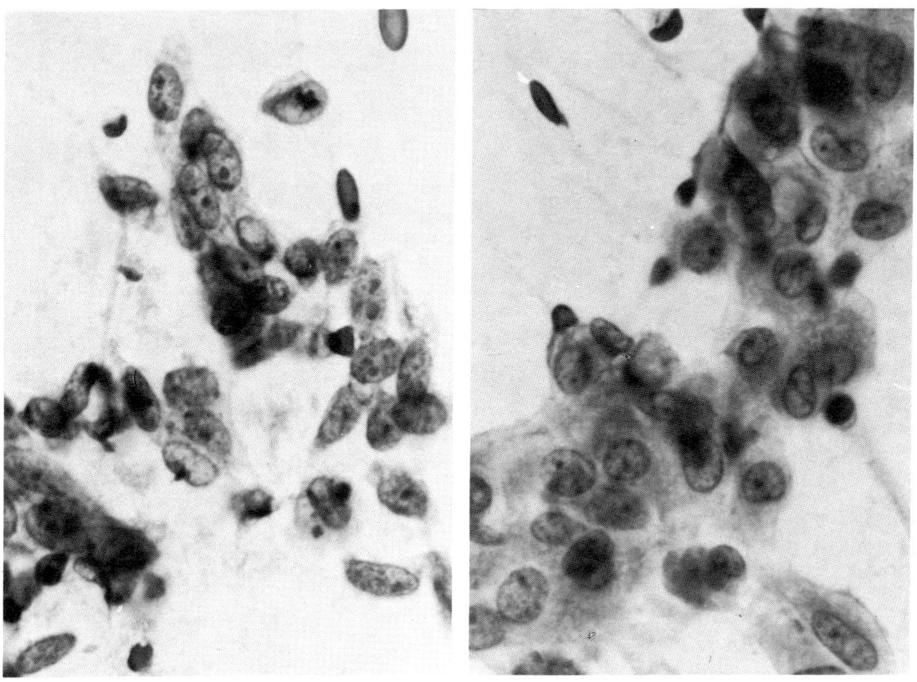

A B

Figure 7-12. Synovial sarcoma. **A.** Single and clustered spindle-shaped cells. **B.** Sheet of glandular-type cells with abundant cytoplasm and vesicular nuclei. (Papanicolaou ×400.)

Table 7-2. Cytologic Differential Diagnosis of Pleomorphic Tumors

TUMOR	ABC	CYTOCHEMICAL AND IMMUNOCYTOCHEMICAL FEATURES	ELECTRON MICROSCOPIC FEATURES
Fibrous histiocytoma, benign and malignant	Histiocytoid and fibroblastic cells, single Multinucleated giant cells	α-1-antichymotrypsin, + α-1-antitrypsin, +	Histiocytoid and fibroblastic cells
Pleomorphic rhabdomyosarcoma	Pleomorphic cells, single and clustered Cytoplasmic cross-striations, rare	α-1-antichymotrypsin, + Desmin, +; myoglobin, + Skeletal muscle myosin, + Skeletal muscle actin, +	Thin- and thick-banded filaments
Pleomorphic liposarcoma	Pleomorphic cells, single and clustered Vacuolated cytoplasm	Oil red 0, + cytoplasmic vacuoles S-100 protein, +	Fat droplets, cytoplasmic
Malignant melanoma	Single cells Two or three distinct cell populations Melanin Nuclear cytoplasmic inclusions Macronucleoli	Fontana, + cytoplasmic granules S-100 protein, +	Melanosomes and premelanosomes
Biphasic synovial sarcoma	Polygonal epithelial cells Spindled cells	Keratin, + Vimentin, +	Desmosomes Intercellular lumens Microvilli Basal laminae
Epithelioid sarcoma	Pleomorphic polygonal cells, single and clustered	Keratin, + Vimentin, +	Features similar to synovial sarcoma
Leiomyosarcoma, high-grade	Spindled and bizarre cells, single and clustered	Smooth muscle myosin, + Desmin, +	Bundle of microfilaments with focal densities

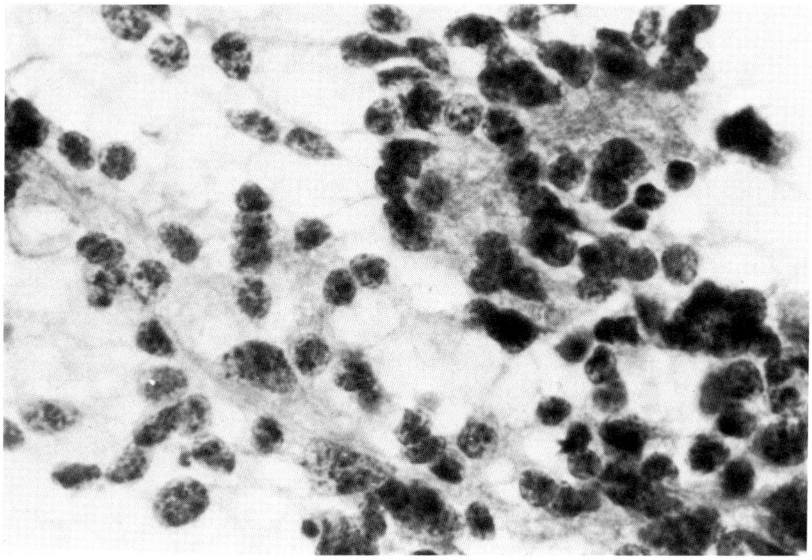

Figure 7-13. Neuroblastoma displaying small round malignant cells with ill-defined cytoplasm singly and arranged in rosettes containing granular material. (Papanicolaou ×400.)

by small round cells with ill-defined and fibrillary cytoplasm, forming rosettes. Macronucleoli are present (Fig. 7-13).

Characteristic cellular features of some round cell tumors are tabulated in Table 7-3.

Metastatic Cancer

Any malignant tumors in the body, except primary cancers of the central nervous system, can metastasize to soft tissue. These include carcinomas of visceral organs, sarcomas, and melanomas. Clinically occult renal cell carcinoma occasionally is diagnosed by its "soft tissue" metastasis. The ABC features of those metastatic cancers are similar to those of their counterparts arising at other sites or organs of the body (see Chapter 6, Metastatic Cancer).

Diagnostic Accuracy and Pitfalls

The cytologic diagnosis of soft tissue tumors is difficult. With an adequate and representative cell sample, however, a correct diagnosis of tumor type may be made. In the majority of cases, it is not difficult to distinguish a benign from a malignant mesenchymal tumor. In experienced hands, a rate of cytodiagnostic

Table 7-3. Cytologic Differential Diagnosis of Round Cell Tumors

TUMOR	ABC	CYTOCHEMICAL AND IMMUNOCYTO-CHEMICAL FEATURES	ELECTRON MICROSCOPIC FEATURES
Extraskeletal Ewing's sarcoma	Single cells	PAS, + PAS-D, −	Glycogen granules, cytoplasmic
Embryonal rhabdo-myosarcoma	Single cells Modest, eosino-philic cytoplasm	*See* Rhabdo-myosarcoma (Table 7-2)	Thin- and thick-banded filaments
Neuroblastoma	Rosettes contain-ing granular, fibrillary material	Grimelius positive cyto-plasmic granules NSE, +	Neurosecretory-type granules
Round cell liposarcoma	Single cells Lipoblasts	Oil red 0, + cytoplasmic vacuoles S-100 protein, +	Fat droplets, cytoplasmic

accuracy of malignant soft tissue tumors by ABC in the range of 85 to 95% has been documented.

Cytodiagnostic pitfalls of mesenchymal tumors are numerous and are due to the complicated histologic patterns of most soft tissue sarcomas. Readers are referred to numerous articles and larger books available.

SUGGESTED READING

Ackerman M, Idvall J, Rydholm A: Cytodiagnosis of soft tissue tumours and tumour like conditions by means of fine needle aspiration biopsy. *Arch Orthop Trauma Surg* 1980;96:61–67.

Golouh R, Us-Krasovec M: Differential diagnosis of the pleomorphic aspiration biopsy sample of nonepithelial lesions. *Diagn Cytopathol* 1985;1:308–316.

Kline TS: *Handbook of Fine Needle Aspiration Biopsy Cytology*, ed 2. New York, Churchill Livingstone, 1988. pp 49–120.

Koss LG, Woyke S, Olszewski W: *Aspiration Biopsy. Cytologic Interpretation and Histologic Bases*. New York, Igaku-Shoin, 1984, pp 422–441.

Lasfield LJ, Anders KH, Glasgow BJ, et al.: Fine needle aspiration of primary soft tissue lesion. *Arch Pathol Lab Med* 1986;110:420–424.

Nguyen GK: What is the value of fine needle aspiration biopsy in the cytodiagnosis of soft tissue tumors? *Diagn Cytopathol* 1988;4:352–355.

Nordgren H, Ackerman M: Electron microscopy of fine needle aspiration biopsy from soft tissue tumors. *Acta Cytol* 1982;26:179–188.

Qizilbash AH, Young JEM: *Guides to Clinical Aspiration Biopsy: Head and Neck.* New York, Igaku-Shoin, 1988, pp 205–264.

Sneige N, Ayala AG, Carrasco CH, et al.: Giant cell tumor of bone: a cytologic study of 24 cases. *Diagn Cytopathol* 1985;1:111–117.

Walaas L, Kindblom L-G: Lipomatous tumors: a correlative cytologic and histologic study of 27 tumors examined by fine needle aspiration cytology. *Hum Pathol* 1985;16:6–18.

White VA, Fanning CV, Ayala AG, et al.: Osteosarcoma and the role of fine needle aspiration. A study of 51 cases. *Cancer* 1988;62:1238–1246.

Willems J-S: Aspiration biopsy cytology of tumors and tumor-suspect lesions of bone. In Linsk JA, Franzen S: *Clinical Aspiration Biopsy Cytology*. ed 2. Philadelphia, Lippincott, 1989. pp 399–420.

8

PROSTATE

The distinction between benign and malignant nodular lesions of the prostate by means of digital examination is difficult and can be erroneous even in experienced hands. NAB for cytologic evaluation of the prostate as an office procedure the first time an abnormality is palpated is widely accepted as a rapid, safe, and reliable method for detecting cancer of the gland. It is more advantageous than the large-bore needle biopsy for histologic diagnosis of prostatic tissue because it samples a larger area of the gland, and it can be repeated several times without causing any serious complications. The NAB is usually performed transrectally with either a Franzen instrument or a 20-gauge, 15-cm long, spinal-type needle attached to a 10-ml syringe. To secure adequate cytologic materials two or three needle passes are required.

INDICATIONS AND CONTRAINDICATIONS FOR NAB

Targets of NAB of the prostate include hard nodules and diffuse enlargement of the gland that are suspected to be malignant. This procedure is also used to grade inoperable prostatic carcinomas prior to hormonal therapy or irradiation. It can detect a recurrent cancer or confirm the nonneoplastic nature of an enlarged prostate. Prostatic NAB is contraindicated in patients with bleeding diathesis and in cases of acute or subacute prostatitis. The latter conditions may cause bacteremia, septicemia and, rarely, death.

BENIGN PROSTATIC ENLARGEMENT

Nodular glandular and stromal hyperplasia of the prostate is prevalent in men over 50 years of age. NAB of the lesion usually reveals a few fragments of benign glandular epithelium. A minimum of three to six groups of these epithelial cells per slide distinguishes the benign from the unsatisfactory specimen. These glandular fragments appear as smooth-bordered monolayered sheets of uniform and polygonal cells in a honeycomb pattern. The individual cells show clear cytoplasm with distinct cell limits, and centrally located nuclei displaying inconspicuous or no nucleoli (Fig. 8-1). A few spindle-shaped myoepithelial cells may be seen at the periphery of large glandular sheets or laying free in the smears. Laminated hyaline round structures (corpora amylacea), inflammatory cells, urothelial cells from the bladder, and fragments of rectal mucosa are not uncommon.

PROSTATITIS

Acute prostatitis. A prostate with acute inflammation is not a target of NAB. Patchy lesions indicative of acute prostatitis may be present in a gland affected by other pathological processes such as nodular hyperplasia or carcinoma. Needle aspiration from such a focus reveals degenerated glandular epithelial cells, necrotic debris, and numerous polymorphonuclear leukocytes.

Chronic prostatitis. A prostate with chronic inflammation may be stony hard on digital examination, and, therefore, it mimics prostatic carcinoma. Aspirate from such a prostate shows necrotic debris, numerous lymphoid cells, macrophages, a

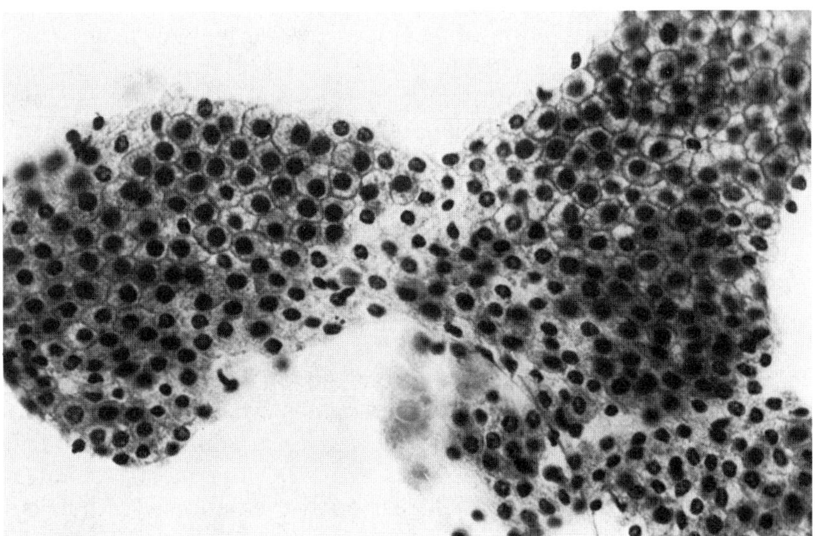

Figure 8-1. Fragment of benign prostatic epithelium showing smooth margins, a honeycomb pattern, and distinct cell borders. (Papanicolaou $\times 250$.)

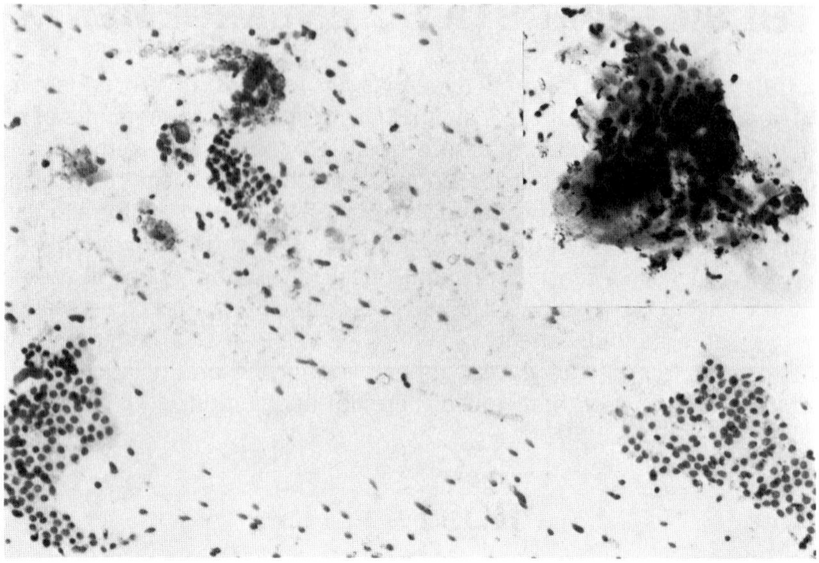

Figure 8-2. Granulomatous prostatitis showing cellularity with benign but edematous epithelial fragments, and inflammatory cells. **Inset:** A multinucleated giant cell. (Papanicolaou ×100.)

few polymorphonuclear leukocytes, and fragments of glandular epithelium with hyperchromatic and enlarged nuclei, and macronucleoli may be present. Cellular dyshesion due to edema may be seen in some glandular fragments.

Granulomatous prostatitis. This condition is usually nonspecific, and it is rarely caused by fungi and mycobacteria. It may occur following the treatment of bladder carcinoma *in situ* with installation of *bacilli Calmette-Guérin*. NAB may be scant in cellularity because of fibrosis. More often, however, it is cell-rich and shows changes similar to those of chronic prostatitis: atypical epithelial cells, necrotic debris, lymphocytes, and histiocytes. The hallmark of the lesion is the multinucleated giant cells and epithelioid cells with carrot-shaped nuclei (Fig. 8-2).

CARCINOMA

Prostatic adenocarcinoma is the most common malignant tumor in men, with the second highest number of cancer-related deaths occurring in patients over 75 years of age. Although there are several grading systems of prostatic carcinoma, the one proposed by Mostofi is most applicable to ABC. In general, aspirates from prostatic carcinomas are cellular and display good correlation with the histologic grades.

Well-differentiated adenocarcinoma. This type of prostatic cancer yields in NAB a cell-rich population of large and small sheets, as well as small groups, of tumor

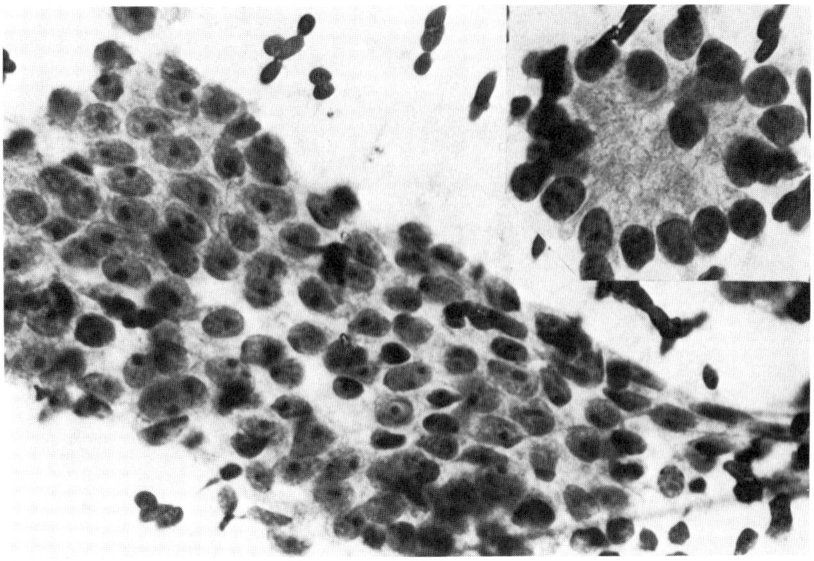

Figure 8-3. Well-differentiated prostatic adenocarcinoma. A fragment of malignant glandular epithelium showing cells with ill-defined borders and macronucleoli. **Inset:** Tumor cells forming a microacinus. (Papanicolaou ×400.)

cells forming microacini that consist of 5 to 10 uniform cells. The epithelial sheets, a number composed of less than 25 cells, have irregular or scalloped margins. The normal honeycomb pattern of those glandular sheets is completely or incompletely effaced. The tumor cell nuclei exhibit mild anisonucleosis with some loss of nuclear polarity. Small nucleoli are present, but macronucleoli are rarely seen (Fig. 8-3). When the cytodiagnosis of a well-differentiated prostatic adenocarcinoma is in doubt, a core needle biopsy is required for histologic evaluation.

Moderately differentiated adenocarcinoma. This tumor shows in aspirates numerous dyshesive cell aggregates and a few single cells. The tumor cells have ill-defined and scanty cytoplasm, and their nuclei are vesicular and slightly irregular with chromatin clumping. Macronucleoli are usually present (Fig. 8-4).

Poorly differentiated adenocarcinoma. Aspirate from this tumor displays numerous malignant cells, which are commonly seen singly and rarely in loose aggregates. Their cytoplasm is usually scant and ill-defined. The nuclei vary in size and shape and show chromatin clumping and eosinophilic macronucleoli. Naked tumor cell nuclei are abundant in some cases (Fig. 8-5).

Important cytologic features of prostatic adenocarcinoma are summarized in Table 8-1.

Other prostatic cancers are rare and consist of mucus-secreting, oat cell, and metastatic carcinomas. Primary prostatic sarcomas are exceedingly rare.

Mucus-secreting carcinoma is characterized in NAB by malignant signet-ring cells and abundant mucus. The tumor cells stain positively with prostatic acid phosphatase or prostate-specific antigen antiserum. Prostatic oat cell carcinoma is

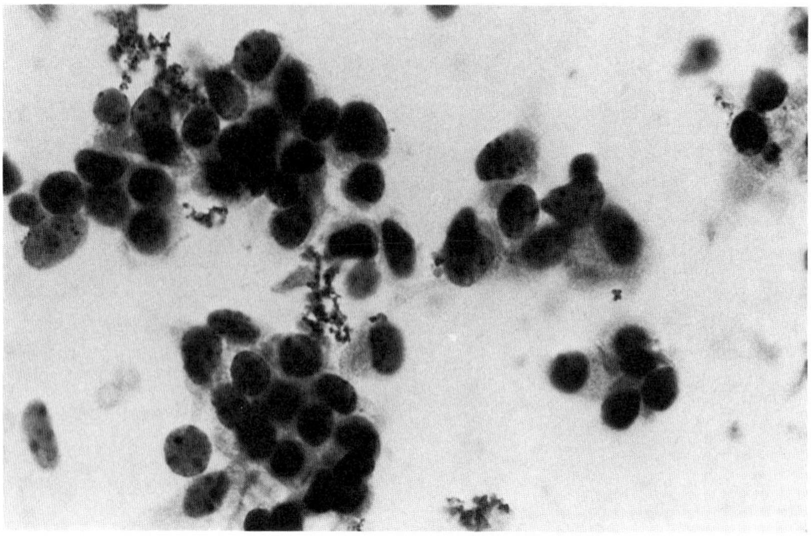

Figure 8-4. Moderately differentiated prostatic adenocarcinoma showing dyshesive small groups of malignant glandular cells with ill-defined cytoplasm, anisonucleosis, and macronucleoli. (Papanicolaou ×400.)

a highly aggressive tumor. Its ABC is similar to that of its counterpart arising from the bronchus.

Secondary tumors of the prostate are usually carcinomas of the bladder and rectum invading the gland. Their aspiration cytologies are similar to those of their counterparts in other locations.

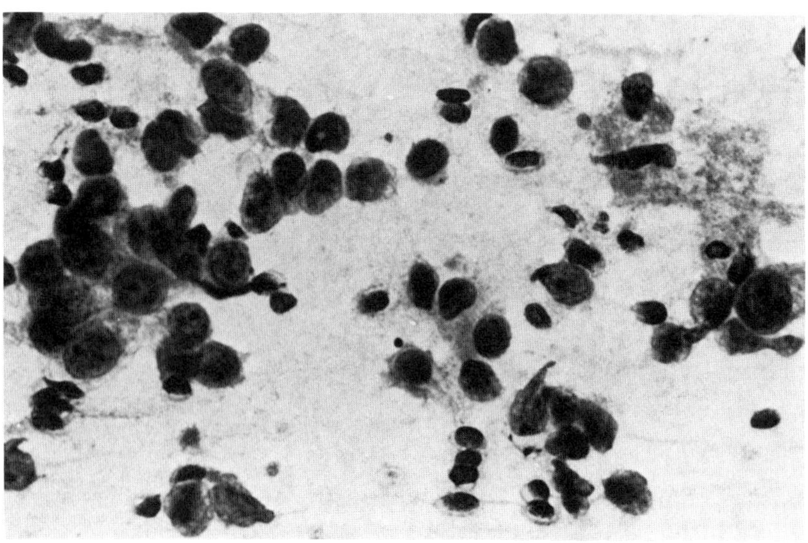

Figure 8-5. Poorly differentiated prostatic adenocarcinoma showing single and loose clusters of malignant cells with scanty cytoplasm, macronucleoli, and naked nuclei. (Papanicolaou ×400.)

Table 8-1. Comparative Cytomorphology of Prostatic Adenocarcinoma and Prostatic Enlargement

ABC	WELL-DIFFERENTIATED CARCINOMA	MODERATELY WELL-DIFFERENTIATED CARCINOMA	POORLY DIFFERENTIATED CARCINOMA	BENIGN ENLARGEMENT
Cellularity	+++	+++	+++	+
Cell arrangement				
Dyshesive sheets and groups of <25 cells	++	+++	+++	±
Honeycomb pattern	Vague	Absent	Absent	Prominent
Single cells	±	+	+++	−
Microglandular complex	+++	++	+	−
Crowding and pilling	++	+	±	±
Anisonucleosis	±	++	+++	±
Macronucleoli	±	+	+	−

CELLULAR CHANGES DUE TO HORMONAL THERAPY

Estrogen administration to patients with prostatic adenocarcinoma may induce regression and disappearance of cancer cells within the gland and in metastasis. Its mode of action is not completely known. However, degeneration and necrosis of tumor cells have been documented. The prostate shows benign squamous metaplasia that can be appreciated in needle aspirate of treated patients.

It has been shown that the presence of glycogenic and metaplastic squamous cells in aspirates of a prostatic adenocarcinoma treated with estrogen is evidence for good response to the treatment. However, this result is not reproducible by other investigators.

DIAGNOSTIC ACCURACY AND PITFALLS

With adequate cytologic material, a diagnostic accuracy of prostatic carcinoma of greater than 90% may be obtained in experienced hands. There are several reasons for a false-negative result. They include the lack of experience of the cytopathologist, the small size of the tumor that escapes the biopsy needle, and the similarity between cells of a well-differentiated prostatic adenocarcinoma and those of a hyperplastic gland. The cell-rich material and the presence of microacini are more characteristic for a carcinoma. Cells of a poorly differentiated adenocarcinoma

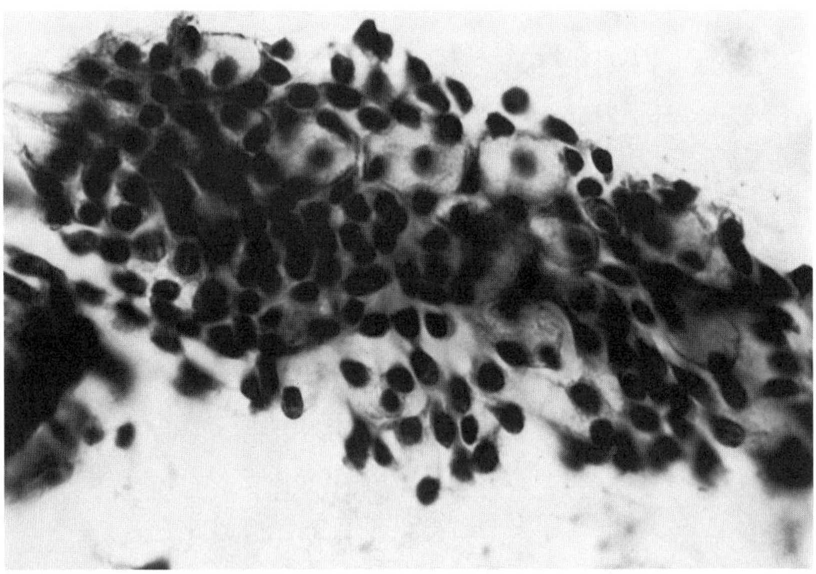

Figure 8-6. Fragments of benign rectal epithelium showing intracytoplasmic mucus. (Papanicolaou ×250).

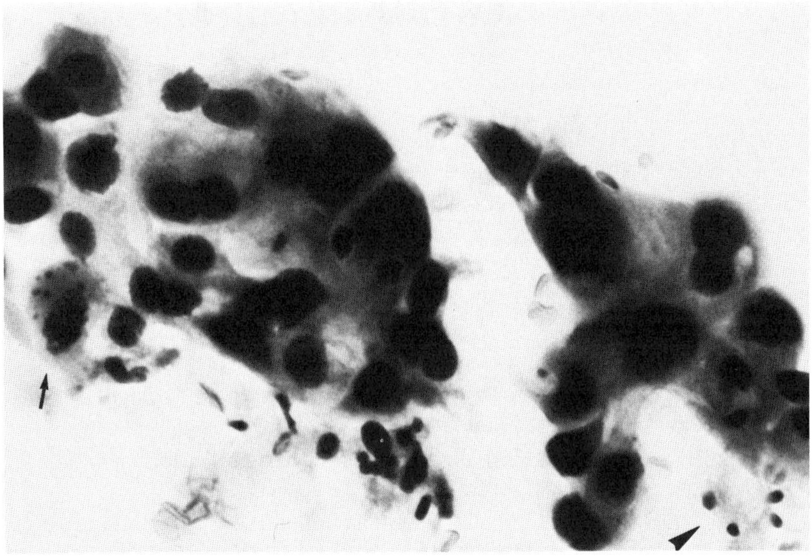

Figure 8-7. Seminal vesicle cells in clusters showing large and hyperchromatic nuclei. One cell shows intracytoplasmic yellow and brown granules (*arrow*). A few spermatozoa are noted (*arrowhead*). (Hematoxylin and eosin ×400.)

may be similar to lymphoma cells. Identification of a few dyshesive clusters of tumor cells showing macronucleoli and lacking nuclear indentations or protusions usually indicates a poorly differentiated prostatic adenocarcinoma. A positive cytoplasmic reaction with prostatic acid phosphatase or prostate-specific antigen antiserum constitutes strong evidence that the cells aspirated are of prostatic origin.

Chronic prostatitis may show highly atypical epithelial cells, mimicking those of a well-differentiated prostatic adenocarcinoma. The presence of cell clusters forming microacini and the high cellularity of the aspirate favor the latter. Repetition of the NAB after treatment for the inflammatory condition or a core biopsy for tissue diagnosis should be performed in all cases with a suspicious diagnosis.

Contamination of the aspirate by cells from rectal mucosa and seminal vesicle cells may cause faulty diagnosis. The rectal epithelial cells usually form large sheets and, rarely, small acini resembling those of a well-differentiated prostatic carcinoma. Rectal cells, however, are characterized by tall, slender, eccentrically located nuclei that are arranged in palisade and by intracytoplasmic mucus-containing vacuoles (Fig. 8-6). Cells from seminal vesicles usually display anisonucleosis, nuclear lobulation and hyperchromasia, and macronucleoli. The presence of intracytoplasmic lipochrome granules and spermatozoa in the aspirate are indicative of their seminal vesicle origin (Fig. 8-7). These contaminated cells will stain negatively with prostatic acid phosphatase or prostate-specific antigen antiserum.

Finally, it should be borne in mind that radiation therapy and chemotherapy may induce cellular atypias for a long period of time after treatment. Thus, the presence of a few poorly preserved pleomorphic cells should not be interpreted as evidence of tumor recurrence.

SUGGESTED READING

Ahmed MN: Fine needle aspiration cytology. In *Urinary Tract Cytology*. New York, Thieme, 1987, pp 89–104.

Carter HB, Riehle RA, Koizumi JH, et al: Fine needle aspiration of the abnormal prostate: a cytohistological correlation. *J Urol* 1986;1:294–298.

Esposti PL: Cytologic malignancy grading of prostatic carcinoma by transrectal aspiration biopsy: a five-year follow-up study of 469 hormone treated patients. *Scand J Urol Nephrol* 1971;5:199–209.

Kaufman JJ, Ljung BM, Walther P, et al.: Aspiration biopsy of prostate. *Urology* 1982;19:587–591.

Kline TS: *Guides to Clinical Aspiration Biopsy. Prostate*. New York, Igaku-Shoin, 1985.

Kline TS, Kohler FP, Kelsey DM: Aspiration biopsy cytology. Its use in diagnosis of lesions of the prostate gland. *Arch Pathol Lab Med* 1989;106:136–139.

Linsk JA, Franzen S: Aspiration biopsy cytology of the prostate gland. In *Clinical Aspiration Cytology*, ed 2. Philadelphia, Lippincott, 1989, pp 283–304.

Mostofi FK, Price EB: Tumors of the male genital system. In *Atlas of Tumor Pathology*, series 2. Washington, DC, Armed Forces Institutes of Pathology, 1973.

9

LUNG, PLEURA, AND MEDIASTINUM

Needle aspiration biopsy for cytologic examination of mass lesions of the lung, pleura and mediastinum now is a routine diagnostic procedure. The NAB can be performed transthoracically under the guidance of image intensification fluoroscopy or under direct vision via a flexible fiberoptic bronchoscope. The former biopsy technique is associated with a high incidence of pneumothorax, which may require a chest tube drainage. This complication is extremely rare in patients who undergo a transbronchial or submucosal NAB performed during a bronchoscopic examination.

INDICATIONS AND CONTRAINDICATIONS FOR NAB

The indications for percutaneous thoracic needle aspiration biopsy and transbronchial needle aspiration biopsy are different.

Transbronchial aspiration biopsy is indicated in patients who are found to have a submucosal tumor or a mass lesion compressing the tracheobronchial tree during bronchoscopy. It is an adjunctival diagnostic method to bronchial brushing and bite biopsy. It may be used to evaluate the submucosal extension of a bronchogenic cancer and to detect its metastasis in peribronchial lymph nodes (cancer staging). It can sample a large submucosal tumor causing a severe bronchial obstruction rendering a bronchial brushing or bite biopsy with forceps impossible. The biopsy needle can go through a large necrotic tumor and sample viable cells for cytodiagnosis. It can also sample a highly vascularized tumor without causing profuse bleeding that may complicate a bronchial brushing or bite biopsy.

Due to the high incidence of pneumothorax, percutaneous biopsy is reserved for patients who have a peripheral mass lesion of the lung that yields no diagnostic cells in sputum, bronchial brushing, bronchial washing, transbronchial NAB, or bronchial bite biopsy materials. This biopsy technique is also used to investigate a pleural or mediastinal mass lesion.

Both percutaneous and transbronchial NABs are contraindicated in patients who have bleeding disorders, pulmonary hypertension, uncontrollable coughing, or intrathoracic hydatid cystic disease. The former also is contraindicated in patients who have advanced emphysema and prior pneumonectomy (see Chapter 2, Complications).

NORMAL LUNG

Normal cellular elements of the lung may be seen in the ABC of a space-occupying lesion located in the thoracic cavity. They consist of ciliated and goblet bronchial epithelial cells, cuboidal cells of the terminal bronchioles, alveolar lining cells, and alveolar macrophages. Fragments of mesothelium or endothelium of large pulmonary blood vessels also may be seen.

The bronchial epithelial cells usually form small groups or clusters or appear singly. These cells are columnar in shape and show a terminal bar with cilia, or contain intracytoplasmic mucous vacuoles (Fig. 9-1). Cuboidal epithelial cells of the

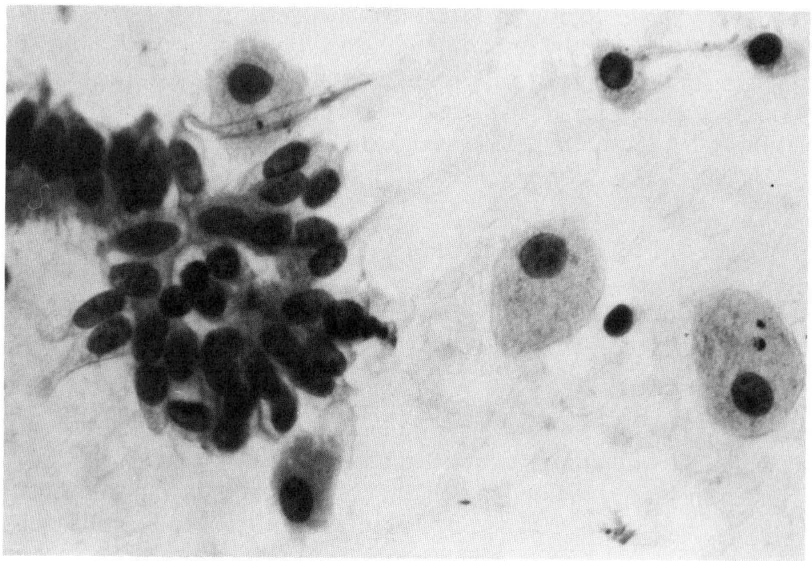

Figure 9-1. ABC of normal lung showing several alveolar macrophages and a fragment of bronchial epithelium. (Papanicolaou ×400.)

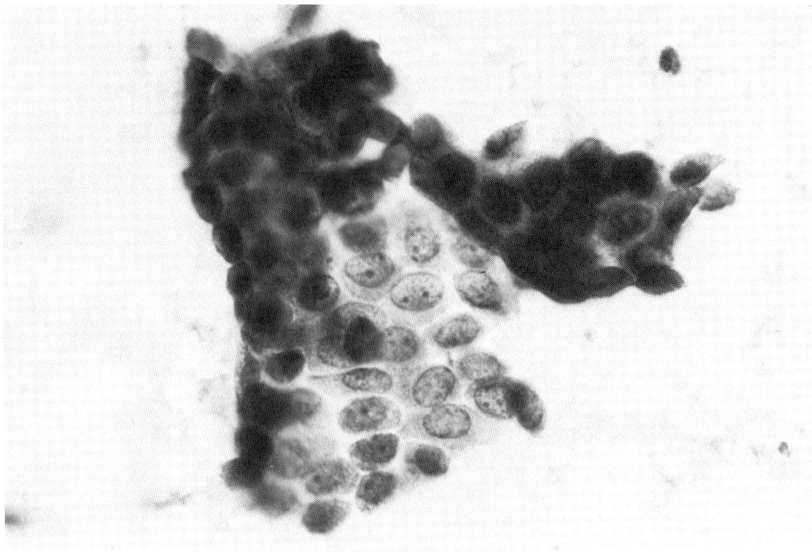

Figure 9-2. A fragment of mesothelium or endothelium. (Papanicolaou ×400.)

bronchioles are most often seen as small epithelial fragments with a honeycomb pattern. Alveolar epithelial cells and alveolar macrophages have a similar morphology. They are polygonal in shape and show vesicular or bean-shaped nuclei. The alveolar macrophages, however, show intracytoplasmic dust particles or foreign body material, and they may be multinucleated. Fragments of mesothelium and endothelium are indistinguishable. They appear as large, irregular, monolayered sheets of cohesive polygonal cells, showing vesicular nuclei with conspicuous nucleoli (Fig. 9-2).

INFLAMMATORY LUNG LESIONS

Pulmonary abscess may develop as a result of an aspiration or bacterial pneumonitis. NAB from the lesion reveals purulent material containing necrotic debris and numerous polymorphonuclear leukocytes.

Tuberculomas in adults usually occur in lung apexes. They may mimic a lung tumor radiologically. NAB from a newly formed tuberculoma shows necrotic debris, epithelioid cells, and multinucleated Langerhans giant cells, as well as numerous young fibroblasts (Fig. 9-3). Commonly, only debris and polymorphic inflammatory cells are seen. Acid-fast bacilli can be demonstrated in smears stained with Ziehl-Neelsen technique.

Pneumocystis carinii pneumonia usually occurs in immunocompromised hosts. The parasites may be identified in materials obtained by bronchial brushing, bronchioloalveolar lavage, and NAB. The characteristic finding is the presence of acidophilic, foamy, granular amorphous materials. This material contains oval or cres-

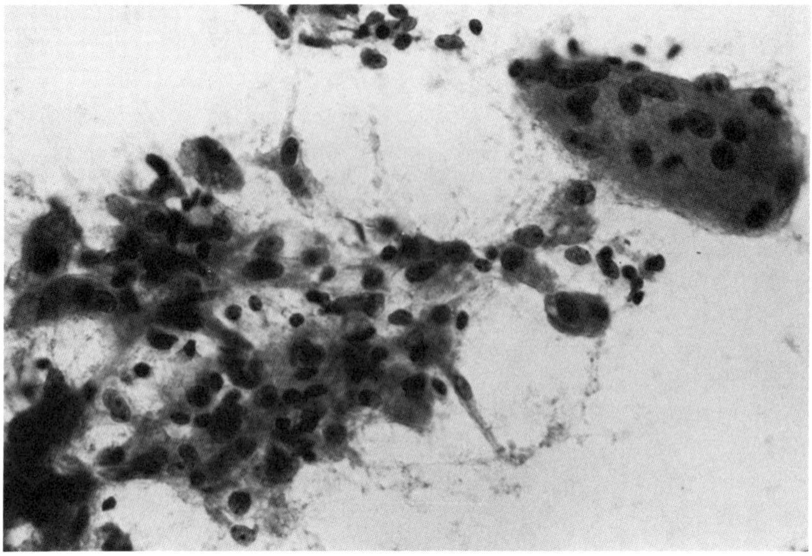

Figure 9-3. Tuberculoma showing a large multinucleated Langerhans cell and several epithelioid cells. (Papanicolaou ×250.)

cent-shaped, 2- to 3-μm cysts with a thick capsule and prominent inner body, which are well-demonstrated by Grocott's methenamine silver stain (Fig. 9-4).

Hydatid cysts may be found in the lung. NAB of an unsuspected cyst may detect hooklets and scoleces characteristic of *Ecchynococcus granulosus* (Fig. 9-5).

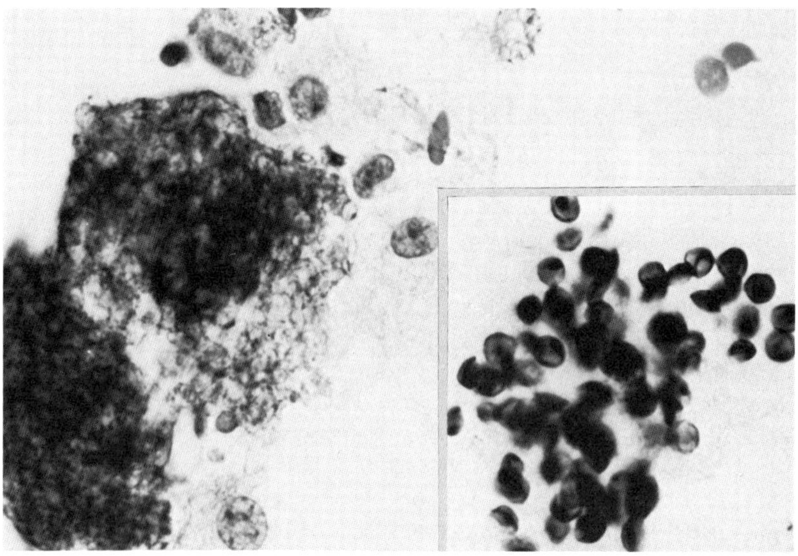

Figure 9-4. Pneumocystis cariini pneumonia showing characteristic foamy eosinophilic material. **Inset:** Parasites with typical features (Papanicolaou ×250, **Inset:** GMS ×400.)

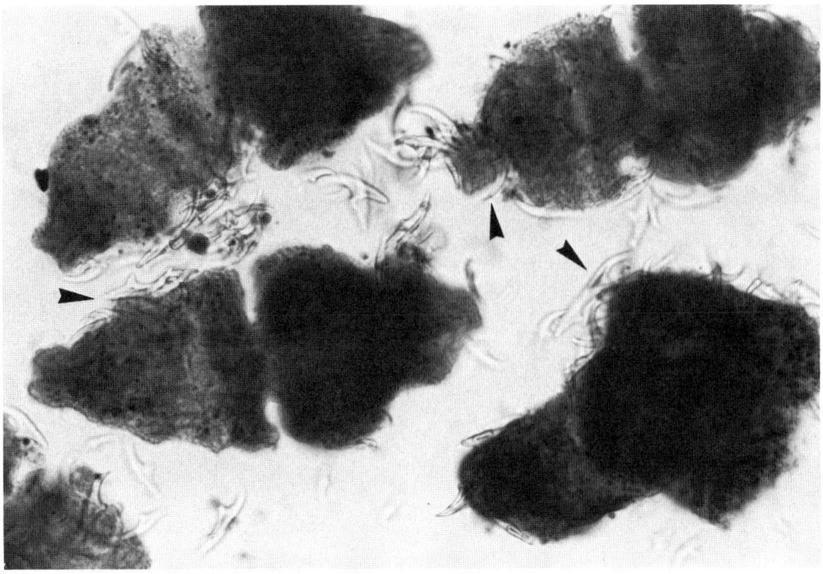

Figure 9-5. Hydatid cyst showing scoleces and hooklets (*arrowhead*) of *Ecchynococcus granulosus*. (Papanicolaou ×250.)

Pulmonary mycoses with granulomatous inflammation may be caused by pathogenic fungi such as *Histoplasma capsulatum*, *Coccidioides immitis*, *Cryptococcus neoformans*, and *Blastomyces dermatitidis*. The incidence of these fungal infections shows great geographic variation, with *Histoplasmosa* endemic in the Middle West, *Coccidioides* in

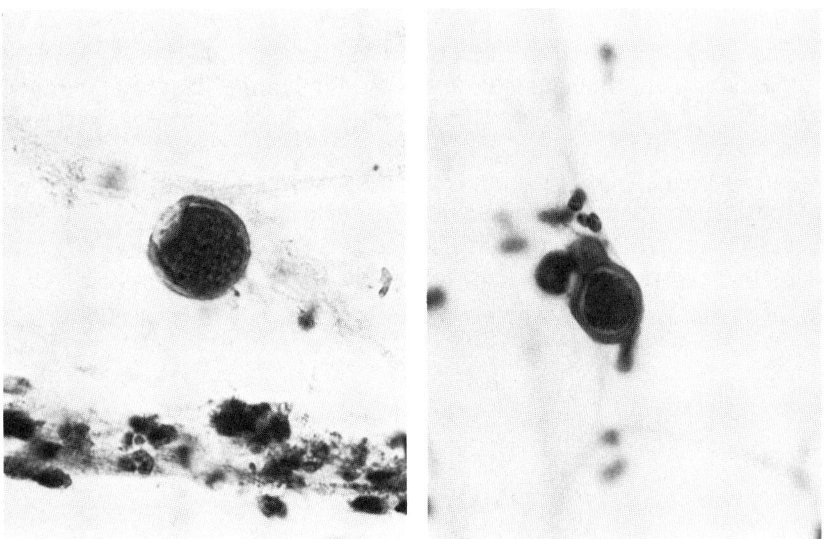

A B

Figure 9-6. Fungal elements. **A.** *Coccidioides immitis* showing a large spherule with thick capsule containing numerous spores. **B.** *Blastomyces dermatitidis* showing the broad-based bud. (Papanicolaou ×400.)

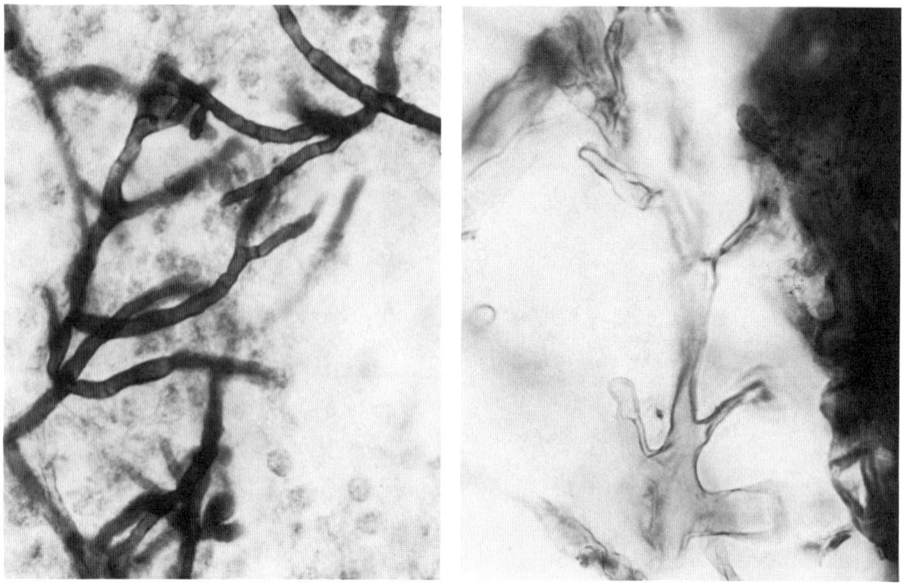

A B

Figure 9-7. Fungal elements. **A.** *Aspergillus fumigatus* showing septate hyphae with 45° branching. **B.** Phycomyces showing ribbon-like nonseptate hyphae with haphazard or 90° branching (**A.** GMS ×400; **B.** Papanicolaou ×400.)

the Southwest, and *Blastomyces* in the Southeast of the United States. Cryptococcosis is ubiquitous and affects patients with debilitating diseases. Patients with uncontrolled diabetes mellitus, chemotherapy for malignant diseases, and HIV infection may be invaded by opportunistic fungi such as elements of *Aspergillus*, *Mucor*, and *Candida* species. Although these organisms tend to occur as disseminated forms in immunocompromised hosts, they may appear as "coin" lesions and are targets of NAB. NAB of those fungal lesions may reveal macrophages, inflammatory cells and necrotic debris, etc., as well as characteristic microorganisms that can be seen with the Papanicolaou staining as well as methenamine silver and periodic acid-Schiff stains (Figs. 9-6–9-8). Table 9-1 summarizes the morphologic features of these fungi.

HAMARTOMA

Hamartoma is the commonest benign neoplasm of the lung. It usually appears as a "coin" lesion and yields in NAB fragments of cartilaginous tissue, loose fibrous tissue, and clusters of benign cuboidal epithelial cells (Fig. 9-9).

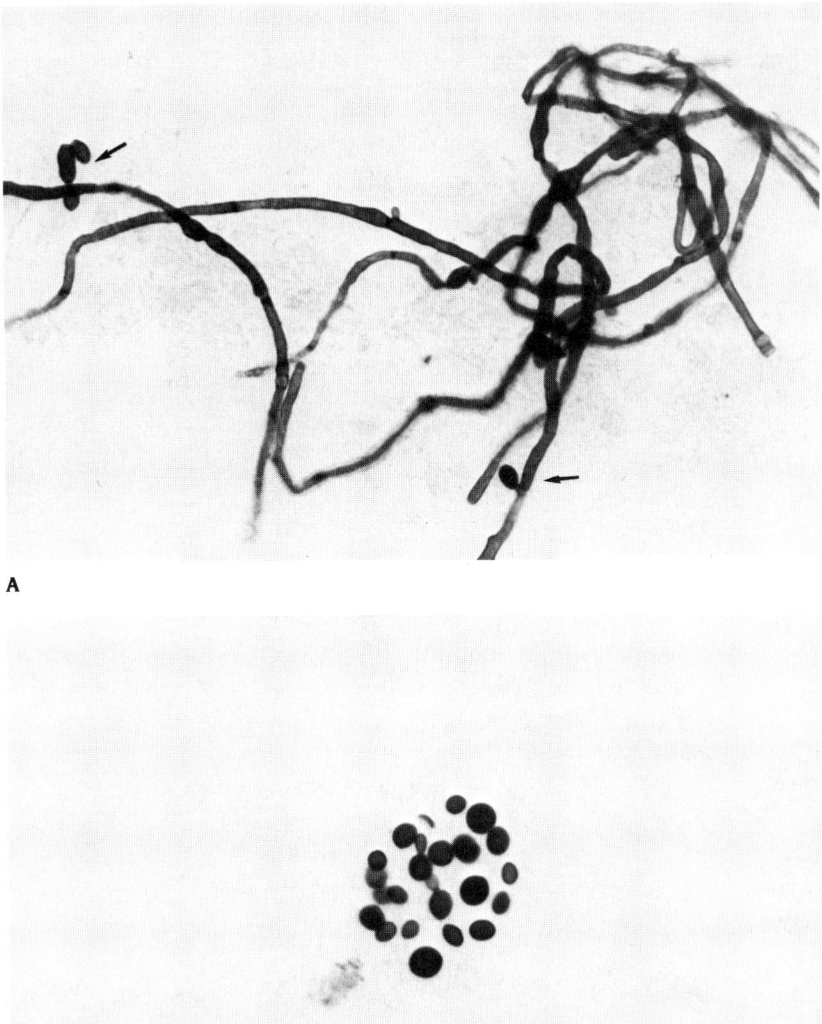

A

B

Figure 9-8. Fungal element. **A.** *Candida albicans* showing pseudohyphae and budding yeasts (*arrow*). **B.** *Cryptococcus neoformans* showing budding with narrow base. (GMS: **A.** ×400; **B.** ×800.)

Table 9-1. Morphologic Features of Pathologic and Opportunistic Fungi

ORGANISM	YEAST OR SPORE	HYPHAE	PSEUDOHYPHAE
Histoplasma	3-μm oval budding yeast Single nucleus with perinuclear clear zone (within macrophage)	–	–
Blastomyces	8- to 15-μm round budding yeast with large base	–	–
Coccidioides	30- to 60-μm spherules with 2–5 micron endospores Thick wall spherules Endospores, no budding	–	–
Cryptococcus	4- to 7-μm round budding yeast with narrow base; Extracellular clear zone	–	–
Aspergillus	–	3- to 5-μm-wide septate hyphae with dichotomous, 45° branching	–
Mucor	–	10- to 15-μm-wide nonseptate hyphae with haphazard or 90° branching	–
Candida	3- to 4-μm round or oval budding yeast	–	+ (Nonbranching)

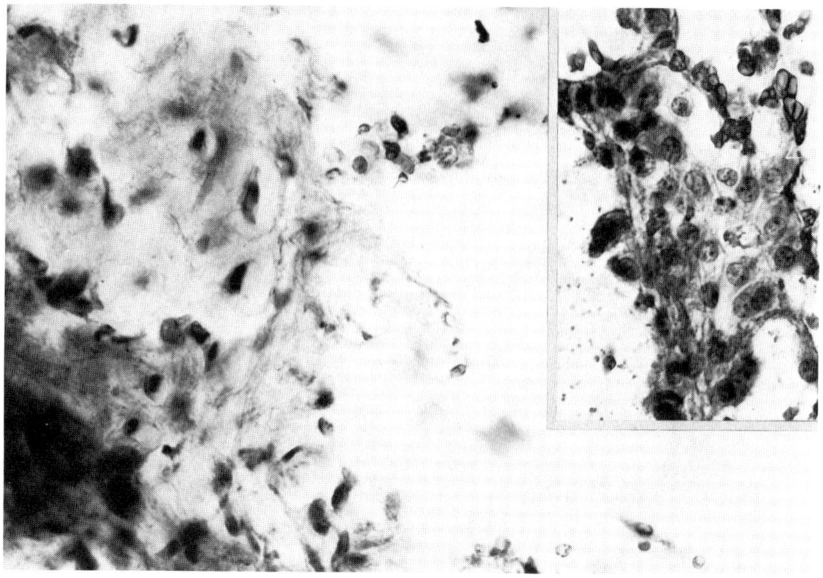

Figure 9-9. Hamartoma showing chondrocytes and fibroblasts. **Inset:** Clusters of benign-appearing epithelial cells. (Papanicolaou ×250.)

MALIGNANT TUMORS OF THE LUNG

Bronchogenic Carcinoma

Bronchogenic carcinomas do not rarely show features of several histologic types, e.g., squamous, glandular, or oat cell carcinomas.

Squamous cell carcinomas constitute about 40% of all lung cancers. About 90% of them arise from large bronchi and are centrally located. Rarely, they appear as a peripheral nodule. The tumor is classified histologically as well- or poorly differentiated. NAB from a well-differentiated squamous carcinoma reveals single and loosely clustered malignant keratinizing cells (Fig. 9-10). A poorly differentiated tumor yields sheets or syncytia of malignant nonkeratinizing squamous cells with scant ill-defined cytoplasm and central nuclei (Fig. 9-11).

Adenocarcinomas of the lung usually occur peripherally and constitute about 20% of all lung cancers. They can be classified as well- and poorly differentiated types. NAB from a well-differentiated tumor reveals fairly regular malignant cells in clusters with focal acinar arrangement. The tumor cell cytoplasm is ill-defined and vacuolated, and it contains mucin. The eccentric nuclei are round or vesicular and show chromatin clumping and macronucleoli (Fig. 9-12). A poorly differentiated tumor yields single and loosely clustered pleomorphic malignant glandular cells.

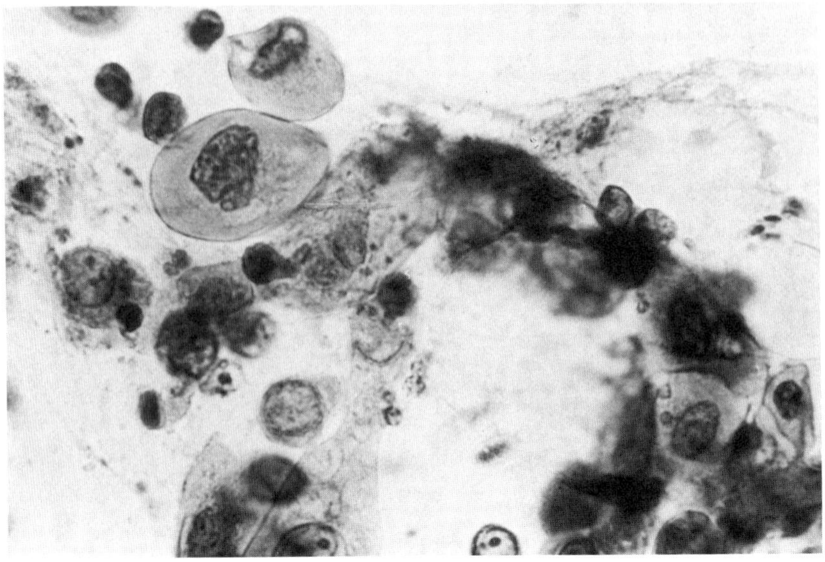

Figure 9-10. Well-differentiated squamous carcinoma showing single and loosely clustered keratinizing tumor cells. (Papanicolaou ×500.)

Bronchioloalveolar cell carcinoma is a histologic variant of pulmonary adenocarcinoma. The tumor can be classified as secretory or nonsecretory, depending on its ability to produce mucin. NAB of a secretory tumor yields irregular tight clusters of uniform malignant glandular cells with vacuolated cytoplasm in a mucoid background (Fig. 9-13). Monolayered sheets and papillary clusters of nonvacuolated

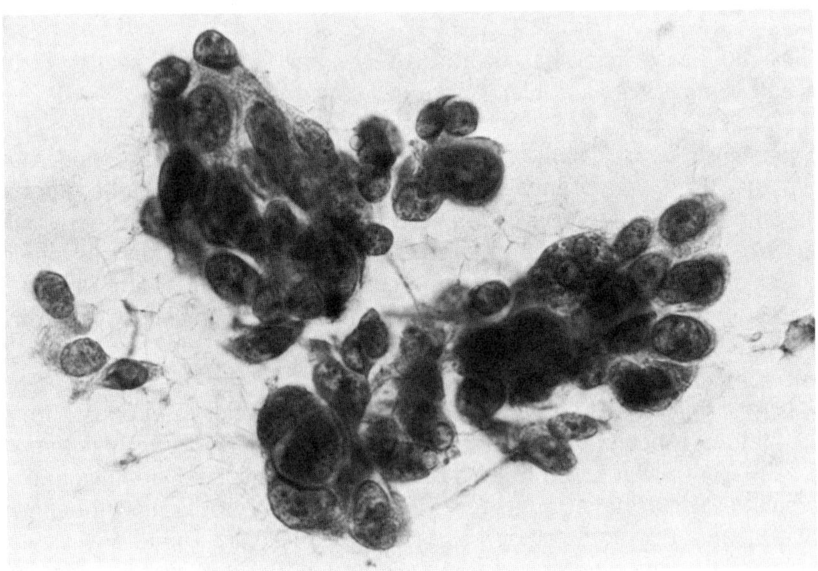

Figure 9-11. Poorly differentiated squamous carcinoma showing a syncytial cluster of nonkeratinizing tumor cells. (Papanicolaou ×400.)

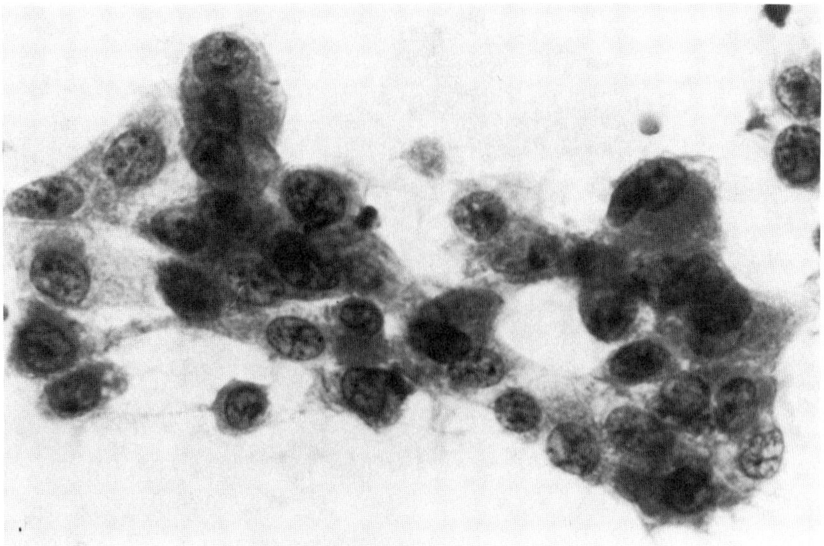

Figure 9-12. Well-differentiated adenocarcinoma showing a group of malignant glandular cells with vacuolated cytoplasm and eccentric nuclei with macronucleoli. (Papanicolaou ×400.)

glandular epithelium with relatively bland nuclei showing nucleoli are seen in the ABC of a nonsecretory tumor (Fig. 9-14).

Large-cell anaplastic carcinomas of the bronchial tree are more commonly located at the periphery of the lung and constitute about 20% of all lung cancers. The

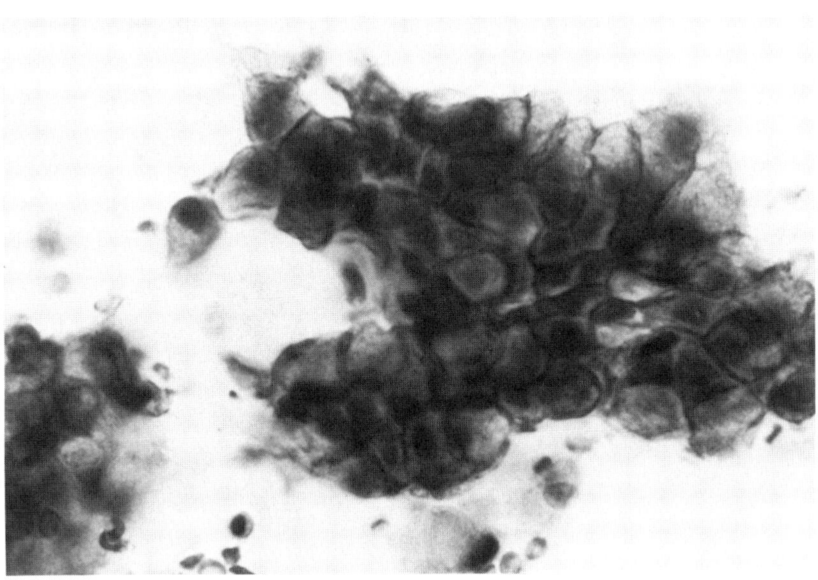

Figure 9-13. Secretory bronchoalveolar carcinoma showing irregular monolayered sheets of tumor cells with vacuolated cytoplasm and eccentrically located nuclei. (Papanicolaou ×250.)

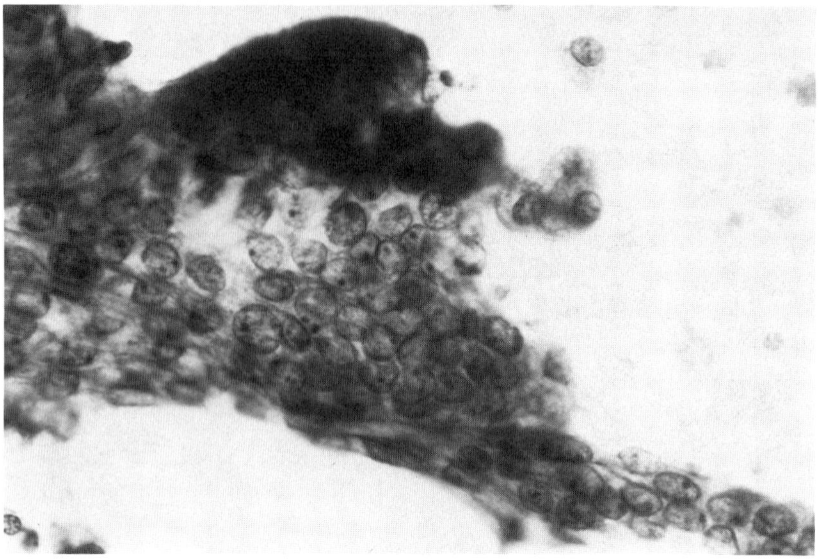

Figure 9-14. Nonsecretory broncholoalveolar carcinoma showing a fragment of neoplastic epithelium without vacuolated cytoplasm and regular nuclei with macronucleoli. (Papanicolaou ×250.)

NAB reveals single and loose groups of malignant cells without squamous or glandular differentiation (Fig. 9-15). Giant cell carcinoma is an aggressive and somewhat unusual variant. It yields in NAB loose groups of pleomorphic, large multinucleated cancer cells (Fig. 9-16).

Small cell anaplastic carcinomas often arise from large bronchi and constitute about 15 to 20% of all malignant lung tumors. Rarely, the tumors are peripherally

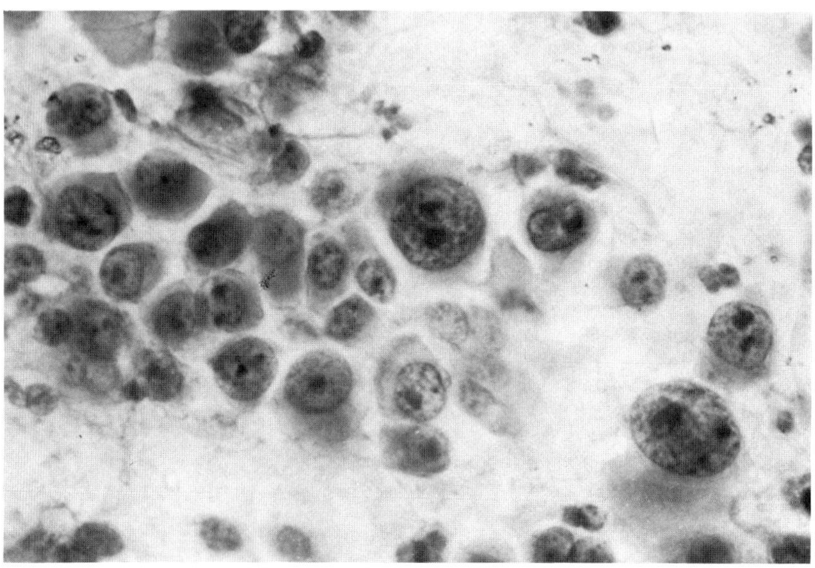

Figure 9-15. Large cell anaplastic carcinoma showing single large pleomorphic cancer cells with macronucleoli. (Papanicolaou ×400.)

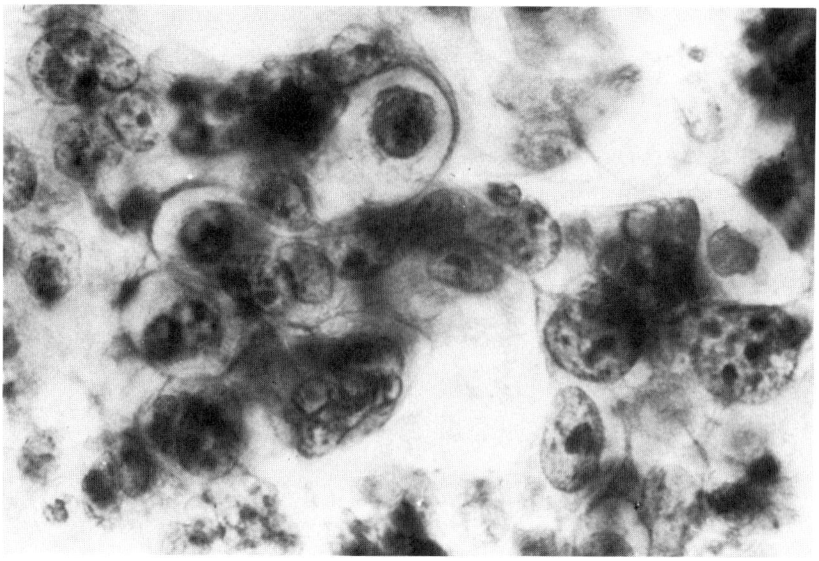

Figure 9-16. Giant cell carcinoma showing pleomorphic and multinucleated neoplastic cells. (Papanicolaou ×400.)

located and appear as a "coin" lesion. Histologically, they are classically subdivided into two morphologic types: oat cell and intermediate cell types. Usually, the tumors are composed of both cell types. NAB shows single and loosely clustered small cancer cells with nuclear molding and a finely granular chromatin pattern. Inconspicuous nucleoli are commonly seen (Fig. 9-17). Basophilic nuclear debris in the form of linear strings is common.

Cellular features of major types of bronchogenic carcinoma are summarized in Table 9-2.

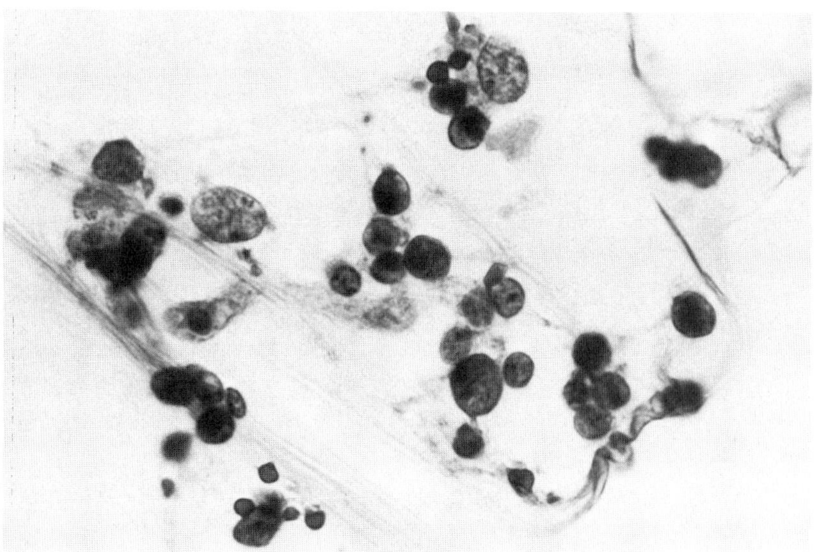

Figure 9-17. Oat cell carcinoma showing single and clustered tumor cells with nuclear molding, and background debris. (Papanicolaou ×400.)

Table 9-2. Comparative Cytomorphology of Major Bronchogenic Carcinomas

ABC	SQUAMOUS CELL CARCINOMA	ADENOCARCINOMA	BRONCHIOLOALVEOLAR CELL CARCINOMA	LARGE CELL ANAPLASTIC CARCINOMA	OAT CELL CARCINOMA
Cell arrangement	Singly Syncytia	Acini Aggregates	Sheets Papillary clusters	Singly Aggregates	Singly Molded clusters
Cell features					
Configuration	Pleomorphic	Columnar	Columnar Cuboidal	Polygonal	Oval
Cytoplasm	Well-defined, keratinized Ill-defined, scant	Vacuolated Scant	Granular Vacuolated	Variable	Scant
Nucleus	Central Bizarre Hyperchromatic	Eccentric Oval Chromatin clumping	Central, eccentric Oval Fine chromatin	Central, eccentric Oval Chromatin clumping	Central Oval Granular chromatin
Nucleolus	Variable	Macronucleolus Often multiple	Variable	Macronucleolus Often multiple	Small
Diathesis					
Necrotic debris	++	+	±	+	+ (Crush artefact)
Mucus	−	−	±	−	−

Carcinoid Tumor

Carcinoid tumors (bronchial adenomas) constitute about 2% of all malignant lung cancers. They are classified into three types: central, peripheral, and atypical. The central and peripheral carcinoid tumors may display similar histologic patterns and consist of monomorphic cells with round nuclei and fairly well-defined cytoplasm arranged in trabecular, solid, or acinar patterns. The peripheral tumors may totally or partially consist of spindle-shaped cells.

NAB from a classic carcinoid tumor reveals single or loosely clustered tumor cells showing ill-defined cytoplasm and hyperchromatic vesicular nuclei. The cytoplasm stains positively with neuron-specific enolase antiserum and show brown black granules with the Grimelius staining technique (Figs. 9-18 and 9-19).

Atypical carcinoid tumor or grade 1 neuroendocrine carcinoma is a more aggressive neoplasm. It shows in NAB slightly pleomorphic tumor cells that resemble those of a small cell anaplastic cancer. The cells, however, display little or no molding and have vesicular nuclei. Generally, no necrotic debris is seen.

Other Lung Cancers

Primary malignant nonepithelial tumors of the lungs are rare. Metastatic cancers are common, and almost all types of carcinoma and sarcoma can metastasize to the lungs. Their cytopathologic patterns are similar to those of their counterparts arising from or metastasizing to other sites of the body. An accurate cytodiagnosis of a metastatic lung carcinoma may be made by comparing its ABC with the tissue section of a previously resected tumor (see also Chapter 6, Metastatic Cancer, and Chapter 7).

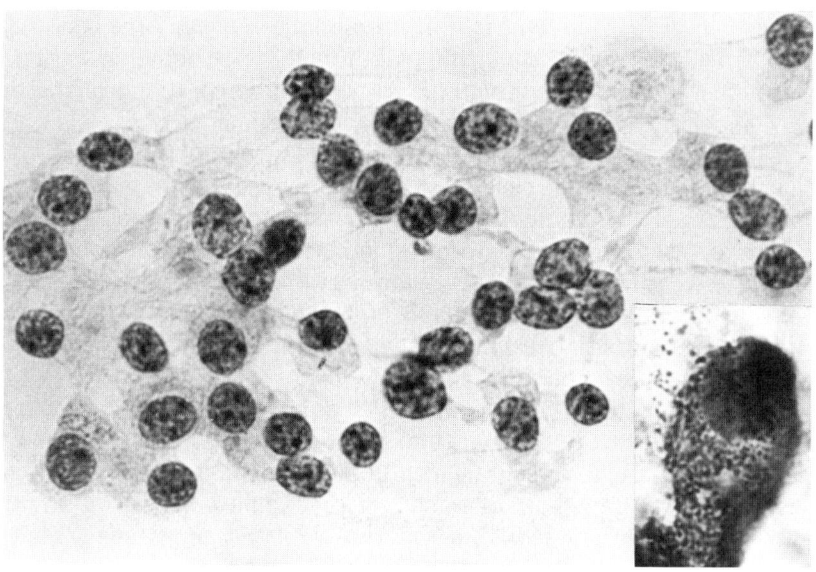

Figure 9-18. Carcinoid tumor showing cells with regular, vesicular nuclei and ill-defined cytoplasm. **Inset:** Intracytoplasmic brown black granules. (Papanicolaou ×500, **Inset** Grimelius ×1000.)

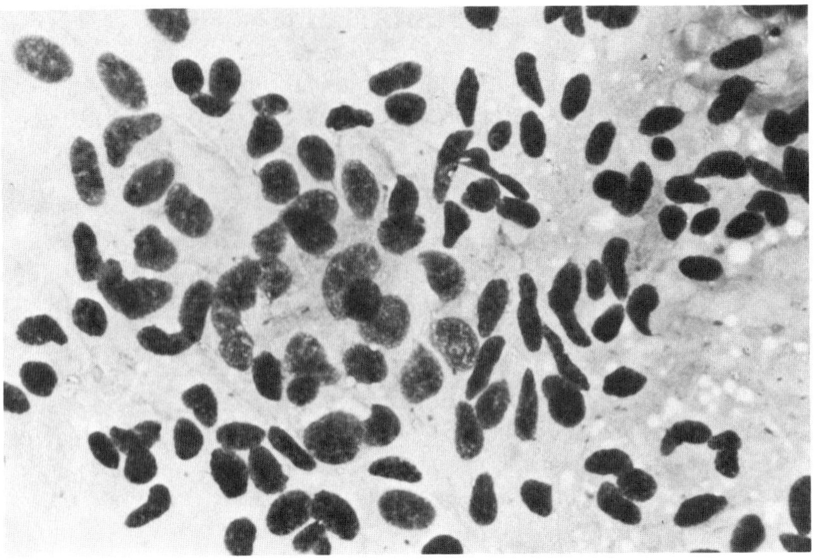

Figure 9-19. Spindle-cell carcinoid tumor showing single and loosely clustered tumor cells. Some tumor cells display oval nuclei. (Diff-Quik ×400.)

DIAGNOSTIC ACCURACY AND PITFALLS

Percutaneous NAB of lung cancers in experienced hands has a diagnostic accuracy within the range of 85 to 90%, in most reported large series. Regarding the tumor typing, the accuracy is about 86% with squamous carcinoma, adenocarcinoma, and oat cell carcinoma cases and is about 70% with large cell anaplastic carcinomas. It should be borne in mind that the cytologic distinction among poorly differentiated squamous carcinoma, poorly differentiated adenocarcinoma, and large cell anaplastic carcinoma can be a diagnostic dilemma.

A false-negative cytodiagnosis of a malignant lung tumor is usually the result of a sampling error. Inadequate cell samples within the ranges of 4 to 18% have been reported, and they occur more commonly with small tumors measuring from 1.0 to 2.0 cm in greatest dimension. Two other important factors contribute to a high false-negative diagnostic rate. These are tumors with extensive central necrosis that yield only necrotic material and no viable tumor cells, and lung cancers associated with a marked desmoplastic reaction that yield scant cell samples inadequate for a confident cytologic diagnosis.

False-positive cytodiagnosis of up to 3% has been reported. The main reasons are the presence of reactive cells with malignant-appearing features that may occur in cases of pulmonary fibrosis and infection. Benign lymphocytic infiltrations also may yield cells simulating those of a small cell carcinoma. Lung cavitation superimposed by infection with *Coccidioides immitis* or *Aspergillus fumigatus* may result in the proliferation of an atypical squamous epithelium lining the cavity; the ABC can be misdiagnosed as malignant squamous cells by inexperienced observers.

Cancer staging errors may occur with transbronchial NAB since aspirates from parabronchial lymph nodes may be contaminated with cancer cells exfoliated in the bronchial secretion. Other sources of error are encountered in patients who undergo chemotherapy and radiation therapy, which produce highly abnormal epithelial cells or mesenchymal cells readily mistaken for cancer cells. Benign lymphoid cells and hyperplastic reserve cells of the bronchial mucosa may mimic cells of a carcinoid or small cell anaplastic tumor.

TUMORS OF THE PLEURA

Benign mesotheliomas are uncommon and vary in size, up to 20 cm in greatest dimension. They are usually localized and are of the fibrous type. NAB of such a lesion reveals only a few benign fibroblastic cells.

Malignant mesotheliomas can be fibrous, epitheliomatous, or mixed in types. About 40% are associated with pleural effusions that may contain diagnostic cells. NAB of a fibrosarcomatous mesothelioma yields single and clustered malignant spindle-shaped cells (Fig. 9-20).

An epitheliomatous malignant mesothelioma yields in NAB isolated, clustered, tight balls of malignant pleomorphic cells with relatively scant ill-defined cytoplasm and large nuclei displaying prominent nucleoli (Fig. 9-21). The tumor cells stain negatively with mucicarmine and carcinoembryonic antigen antiserum and positively with keratin and vimentin antisera. They give a variable reaction to periodic acid-Schiff staining.

Metastatic cancers to the pleura are commoner than primary pleural tumors. Carcinomas or sarcomas arising from any visceral organs or sites may spread to the

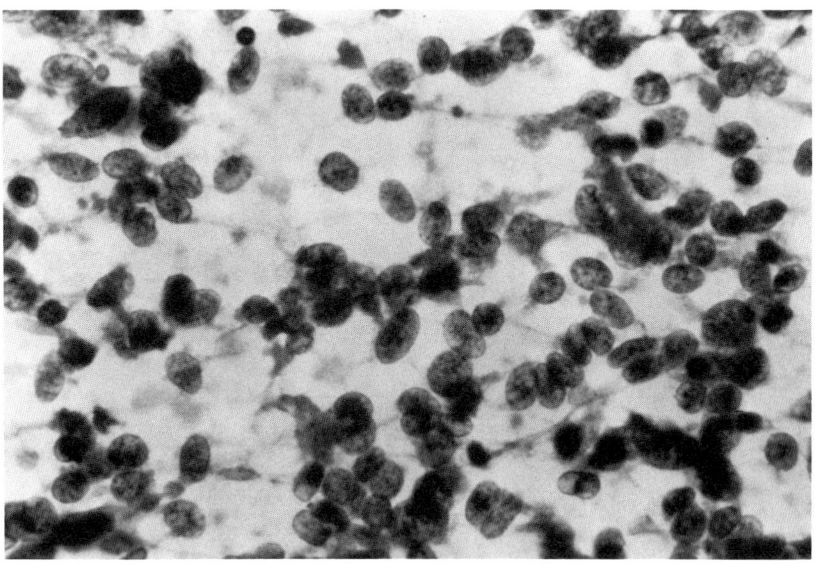

Figure 9-20. Fibrosarcomatous mesothelioma showing single and clustered spindle-shaped cells with ill-defined cytoplasm and oval nuclei. (Papanicolaou ×400.)

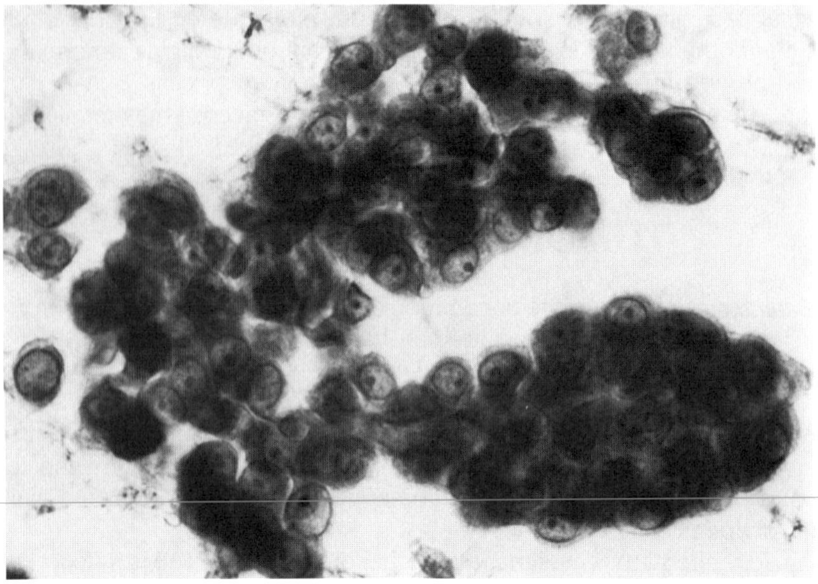

Figure 9-21. Epitheliomatous malignant mesothelioma showing clustered and ball-like groups of tumor cells with scant cytoplasm and macronucleoli. (Papanicolaou ×400.)

pleura, and they are usually associated with pleural effusions containing cancer cells. Their cytologic manifestations are similar to those of the primary tumors of the same histologic types arising from other sites.

The main problem encountered in ABC of an epitheliomatous malignant mesothelioma is the differential diagnosis with a metastatic adenocarcinoma to the lung or pleura. Special stainigs and immunocytochemical studies of the aspirated tumor cells, using selected antisera, may be helpful in this situation. Important cytologic features of adenocarcinomas and epitheliomatous malignant mesotheliomas are tabulated in Table 9-3.

MEDIASTINAL SPACE-OCCUPYING LESIONS

Space-occupying lesions of the mediastinum may be congenital, acquired, or neoplastic in nature.

Mediastinal cysts may be of pericardial, bronchogenic, or enteric origins. The two latter conditions are congenital. NAB of bronchogenic and enteric cysts yields a variable amount of liquid material containing a few single or clustered bronchial epithelial and gastrointestinal epithelial cells, respectively. A pericardial cyst usually is the result of a mediastinal inflammatory process. Cytologic examination of the liquid contents of a noninfected cyst reveals a few fragments of benign mesothelium.

Table 9-3. Comparative Cytomorphology of Malignant Mesothelioma and Adenocarcinoma

ABC	MALIGNANT MESOTHELIOMA	ADENOCARCINOMA
Cell arrangement	Singly Ball-like clusters	Sheets, aggregates, or acini
Tumor cells		
Configuration	Round Polygonal	Round Polygonal Columnar
Cytoplasm	Well-defined Granular	Ill-defined Vacuolated
Nuclei	Oval Macronucleoli Chromatin, fine	Oval Macronucleoli Chromatin, clumped
Other		
Mucicarmine	−	+
Periodic acid-Schiff	±	+
Carcinoembryonic antigen	−	±
Keratin		
Low-molecular weight	+	+
High-molecular weight	+	−
Vimentin	+	±

Germ cell tumors are located mainly in the anterior mediastinum. Seminoma and dysgerminoma are the most common malignant tumors, and benign teratoma is the commonest benign neoplasm. Choriocarcinoma, embryonal carcinoma, and endodermal sinus tumor are rarely found in this location. Benign teratoma is cystic and yields a variable amount of fluid containing keratinous squames. Glandular epithelium of respiratory type may be seen (see Chapter 6, Germ Cell Tumors).

Thymomas can be benign or malignant. They are usually located in the superior mediastinum. Benign thymomas are encapsulated while the malignant ones are characterized by an extensive invasion of the tumor capsule and adjacent structures. NAB from a benign thymoma reveals an admixture of lymphocytes and single or clustered epithelial cells with abundant cytoplasm (Fig. 9-22).

Neural tumors occur almost exclusively in the posterior mediastinum. Neuroblastoma and ganglioneuroblastoma are mainly found in children while ganglioneuroma, neurofibroma, and neurilemoma are seen in adults. Cytomorphologic characteristics of neural tumors are discussed in Chapters 7 and 12.

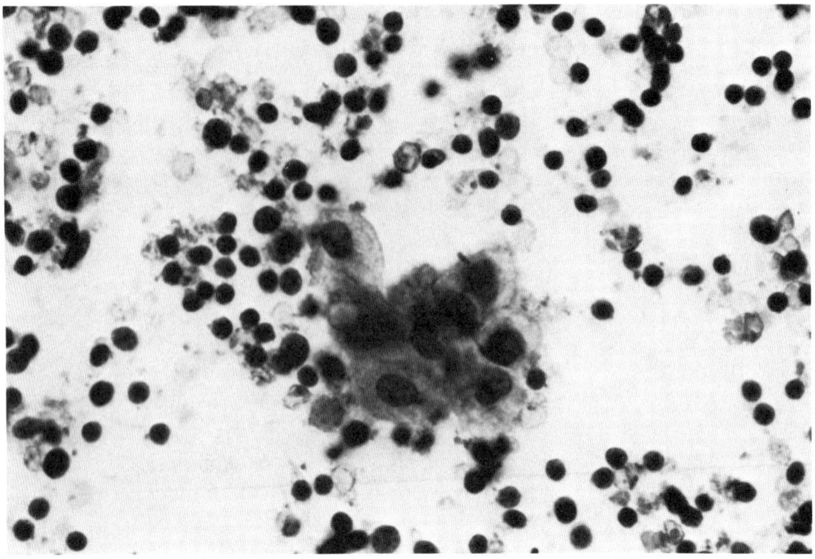

Figure 9-22. Thymoma showing clustered epithelial cells and numerous lymphocytes. (Papanicolaou ×400.)

Other tumors, such as lymphomas, metastatic cancers, and soft tissue tumors of different types, may be encountered in the mediastinum. Of the metastatic cancers, bronchogenic carcinomas are the commonest.

SUGGESTED READINGS

Bhat N, Bhagat P, Pearlman ES, et al.: Transbronchial needle aspiration biopsy in the diagnosis of pulmonary neoplasms. *Diagn Cytopathol* 1990;6:14–17.

Bonfiglio TA: *Cytologic Interpretation of Transthoracic Fine Needle Aspiration Biopsy*. New York, Masson, 1983.

Johnston WW: Percutaneous fine needle aspiration biopsy of the lung. A study of 1015 patients. *Acta Cytol* 1984;28:218–224.

Johnston WW: Cytologic diagnosis of lung cancer. Principles and problems. *Pathol Res Pract* 1986;181:1–36.

Kline TS: *Handbook of Fine Needle Aspiration Biopsy Cytology*, ed 2. New York, Churchill Livingstone, 1988, pp 253–295.

Koss LG, Woyke S, Olszewski W: *Aspiration Biopsy. Cytologic Interpretation and Histologic Bases*. New York, Igaku-Shoin, 1984, pp 287–349.

Nguyen GK: Fine needle aspiration biopsy cytology of metastatic renal cell carcinoma. *Acta Cytol* 1988; 32:409–414.

Rosen S: Mediastinum. In Kline TS: *Handbook of Fine Needle Aspiration Biopsy Cytology*, ed 2. New York, Churchill Livingstone, 1988, pp 297–316.

Rosenthal DL: *Cytopathology of Pulmonary Diseases*. Basel, Karger, 1988.

Tao LC: *Guides to Clinical Aspiration Biopsy. Lung, Pleura and Mediastinum*. New York, Igaku-Shoin, 1988.

10

PANCREAS AND AMPULLARY REGION

The clinical diagnosis of mass lesions of the pancreas and its ampullary region is challenging. Both core needle biopsy and wedge section of pancreatic tissue for histologic diagnosis are associated with a significant risk of morbidity and even mortality, and the tissue samples obtained are quite often unreliable for a morphologic diagnosis of pancreatic cancer because of the often-associated chronic pancreatitis. NAB for cytologic evaluation of the pancreas has proved to be a safe and highly accurate diagnostic procedure. It can be performed intraoperatively or percutaneously under guidance of radiologic imaging techniques. A positive cytologic diagnosis of an inoperable pancreatic mass is an indication for irradiation or chemotherapy, obviating a laparotomy for tissue biopsy.

INDICATIONS AND CONTRAINDICATIONS FOR NAB

The main indication for NAB of the pancreas is the presence of a pancreatic mass lesion that is either palpable or visualized by radiologic imaging techniques. The technique can also be used to confirm or rule out a suspected pancreatic cancer that is well-known to mimic a chronic pancreatitis clinically and at laparotomy. If performed peroperatively, it is also helpful in localizing a small pancreatic neuroendocrine tumor or a cancer of the ampullary region that is not well-visualized by radiologic imaging techniques or by palpation and direct examination at laparotomy.

Pancreatic NAB is contraindicated in patients with bleeding disorders and in patients who are suspected of having intraabdominal hydatid cysts, because the contact of the cyst contents with the peritoneum may cause an anaphylactic shock.

NORMAL PANCREAS

Needle aspirate from normal pancreatic tissue is usually cellular and shows numerous acinar cells and a few fragments of pancreatic ductal epithelium. Fragments of peritoneum or endothelium may also be aspirated. Normal pancreatic endocrine cells are rarely identified.

Ductal epithelium presents as irregular cohesive sheets of columnar or cuboidal cells with a honeycomb pattern. They show regular, round, or oval nuclei with a finely granular chromatin and inconspicuous nucleoli (Fig. 10-1). Nuclei at the free borders of the ductal epithelial fragments may be arranged in palisade. Single columnar ductal cells with foamy cytoplasm are also present.

Acinar cells are seen either singly or in clusters (Fig. 10-2). They are pyramidal in shape and show granular or vacuolated cytoplasm, as well as centrally or basally located round nuclei. The nuclear chromatin is finely granular, and the nucleolus inconspicuous.

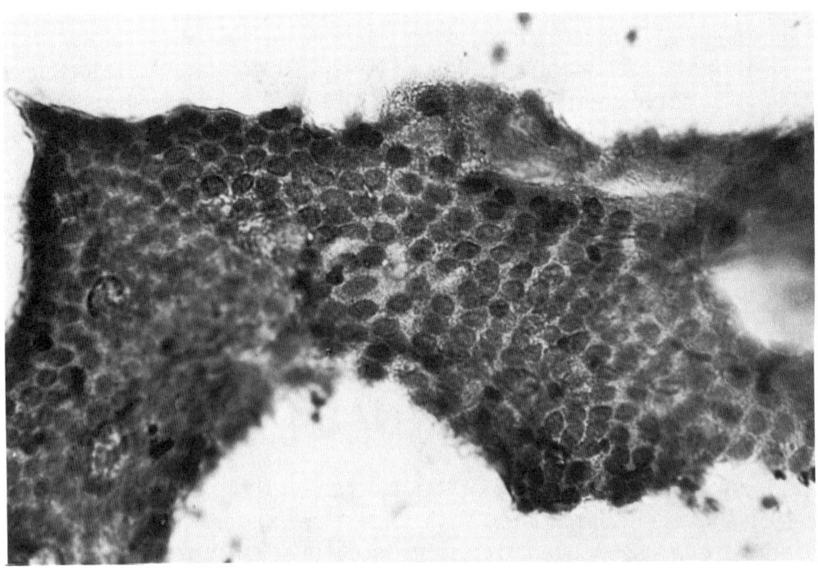

Figure 10-1. Fragment of normal ductal epithelium. (Papanicolaou ×250.)

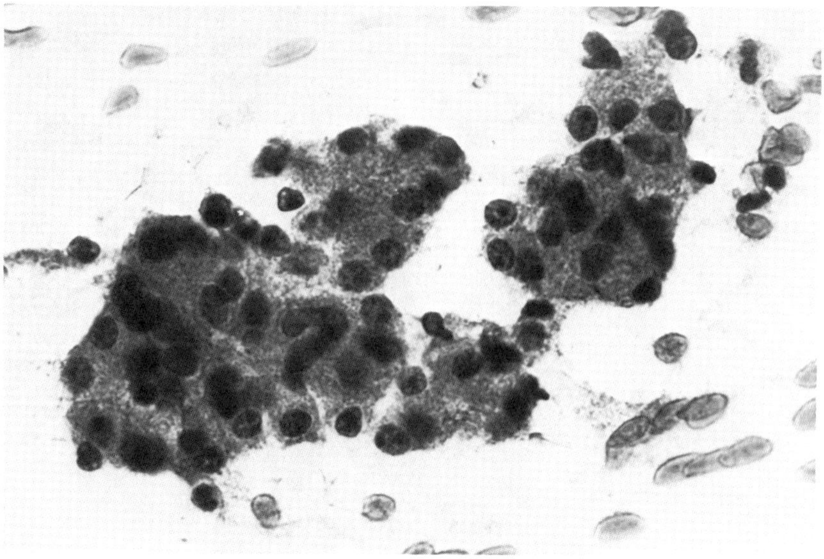

Figure 10-2. Normal acinar cells. (Papanicolaou ×400.)

Pancreatic endocrine cells, when identifiable, are seen as polygonal cells in small clusters. They show pale cytoplasm and round nuclei with inconspicuous nucleoli.

Fragments of endothelium or mesothelium are similar and present as irregular sheets of polygonal cells with ill-defined cytoplasm, round or oval nuclei, and slightly prominent nucleoli. Thin clusters of spindle-shaped fibroblasts of pancreatic interstitial tissue may also be aspirated.

INFLAMMATORY LESIONS

Acute hemorrhagic pancreatitis is a rare target of NAB. Aspirate from an acutely inflamed gland reveals inflammatory exudate, necrotic fat, and degenerated acinar and ductal epithelial cells. Hemosiderin-laden macrophages can be seen at latter stages.

Chronic pancreatitis. In well-established chronic pancreatitis there are extensive fibrosis and loss of exocrine tissue. Focal calcification and nests of hyperplastic pancreatic endocrine cells are not uncommon. Acinar and ductal epithelial cells may display cellular atypias with anisonucleosis and conspicuous nucleoli (Fig. 10-3). There are no particular cellular changes that are diagnostic of a chronic pancreatitis, but the cellular findings usually support the clinical diagnosis. It should be borne in mind that although chronic pancreatitis may be associated with pancreatic carcinoma, hyperplastic endocrine cells may show nuclear hyperchromasia and pleomorphism and may be mistaken for malignant glandular cells (Fig. 10-4).

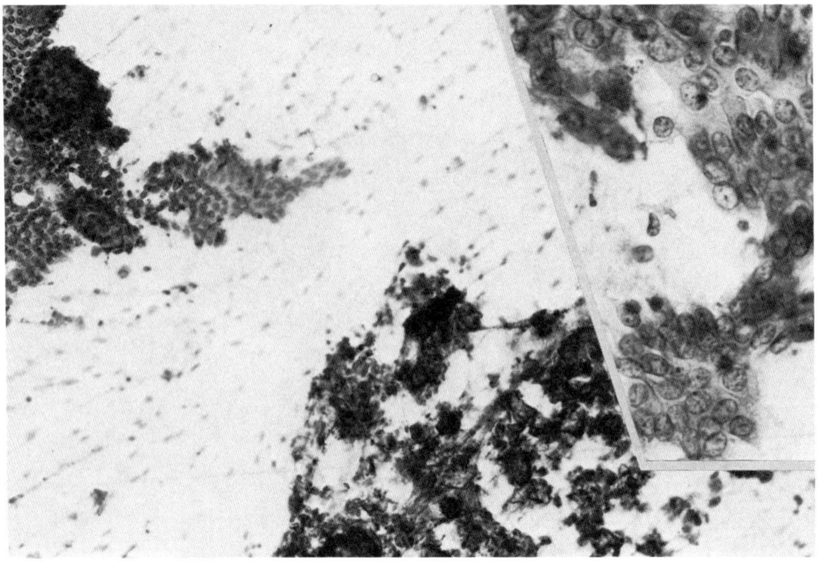

Figure 10-3. Chronic pancreatitis. Large fragment of benign duct epithelium and calcified material. **Inset:** Fragment of atypical ductal epithelium showing nuclear atypia. (Papanicolaou ×100, **Inset** ×250.)

PANCREATIC CYSTIC LESIONS

Pseudocyst of the pancreas. This lesion develops as a late complication of an acute pancreatitis or pancreatic trauma. Aspiration of a clear and watery fluid is

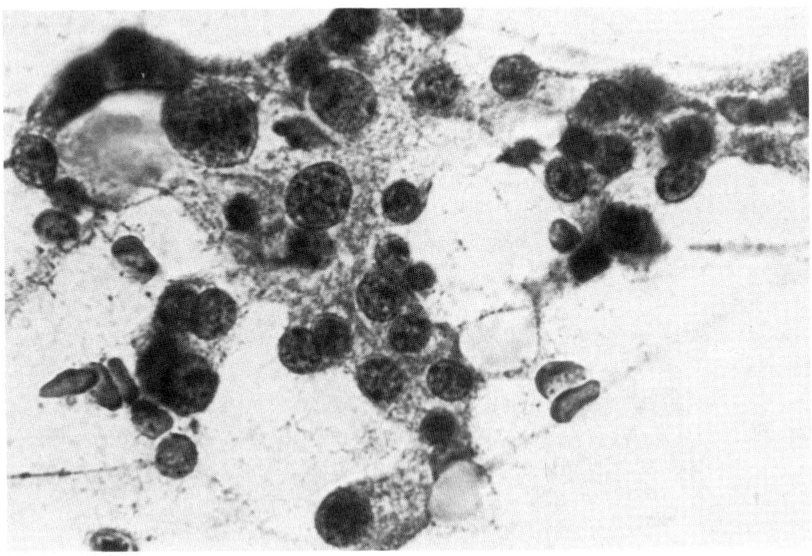

Figure 10-4. Hyperplastic endocrine cells showing hyperchromatic slightly pleomorphic nuclei and granular ill-defined cytoplasm. (Papanicolaou ×800.)

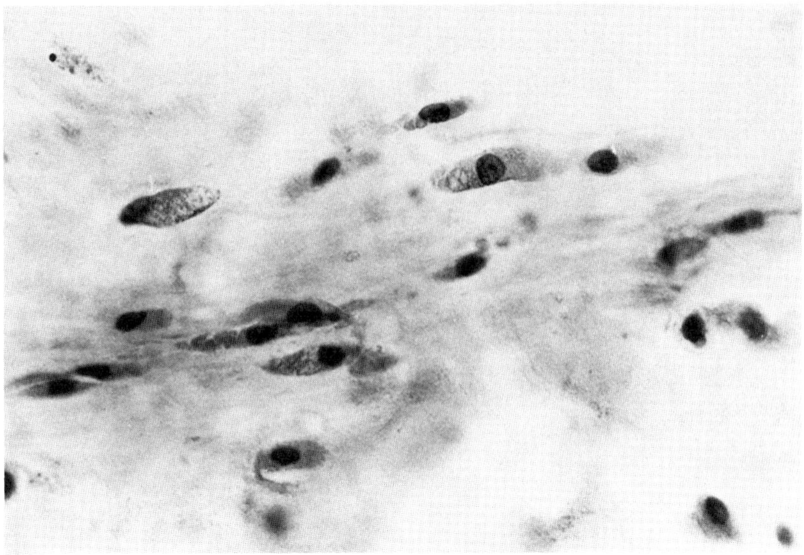

Figure 10-5. Mucinous tumor showing single benign mucus-secreting columnar cells in a mucinous background. (Papanicolaou ×250.)

strongly suggestive of a pancreatic pseudocyst. Microscopic examination of the cyst contents usually reveals a few foamy histiocytes. Necrotic debris and polymorphonuclear leukocytes may be seen if the cyst is infected.

Mucinous cystic lesion of the pancreas is regarded as a malignant or potentially malignant neoplasm. The tumor is usually multilocular, and careful histologic examination of the cyst wall usually detects foci of adenocarcinoma. Cytologic examination of the cyst contents may reveal only benign mucus-secreting cells singly, in clusters, or in sheets (Fig. 10-5). Sheets of bizarre mucus-secreting cells may also be seen.

CARCINOMA OF DUCT CELL ORIGIN

Duct cell adenocarcinoma is the commonest type of pancreatic carcinoma accounting for 75% of all cancers of that organ. Sixty percent of these tumors are located in the head of the gland, and they average 5 cm in diameter when clinically detected. The cancer can be well- or poorly differentiated, but usually a mixed pattern is present. Papillary features are noted in about 10% of cases, and foci of other histologic types may be present in up to 5% of the cases.

The cell-rich aspirate from a well-differentiated duct cell adenocarcinoma reveals single or dyshesive clustered malignant glandular cells with indistinct cell borders, loss of nuclear polarity, and minimal nuclear atypia (Fig. 10-6). The cytodiagnosis of a poorly differentiated duct cell adenocarcinoma is usually easy in a representative sample, because cancer cells are readily identifiable by all criteria of

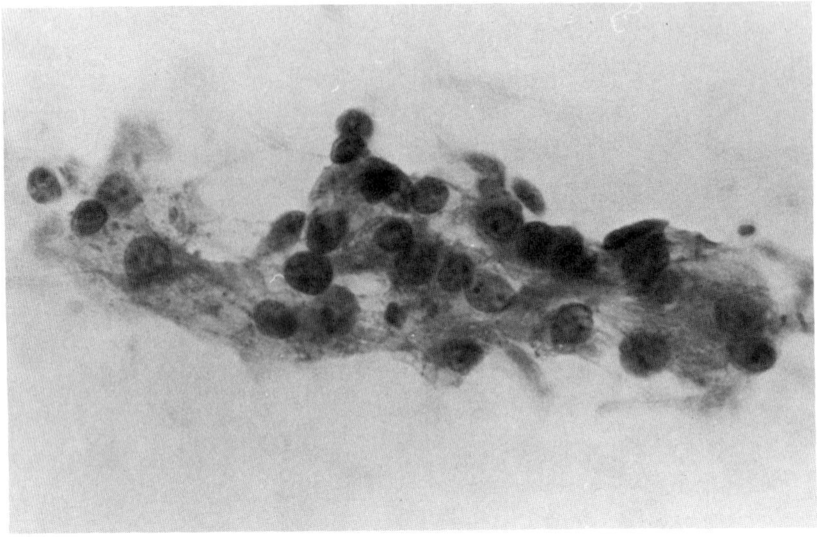

Figure 10-6. Well-differentiated duct cell adenocarcinoma. A dyshesive cluster of indistinctly bordered tumor cells displaying mild nuclear alterations and conspicuous nucleoli. (Papanicolaou ×400.)

malignancy (Fig. 10-7). Three-dimensional papilla-like clusters of tumor cells are usually indicative of a glandular malignancy.

Variants of duct cell carcinoma. Pleomorphic carcinoma, mucinous carcinoma, giant cell carcinoma (osteoclastoid type), adenosquamous carcinoma, and squa-

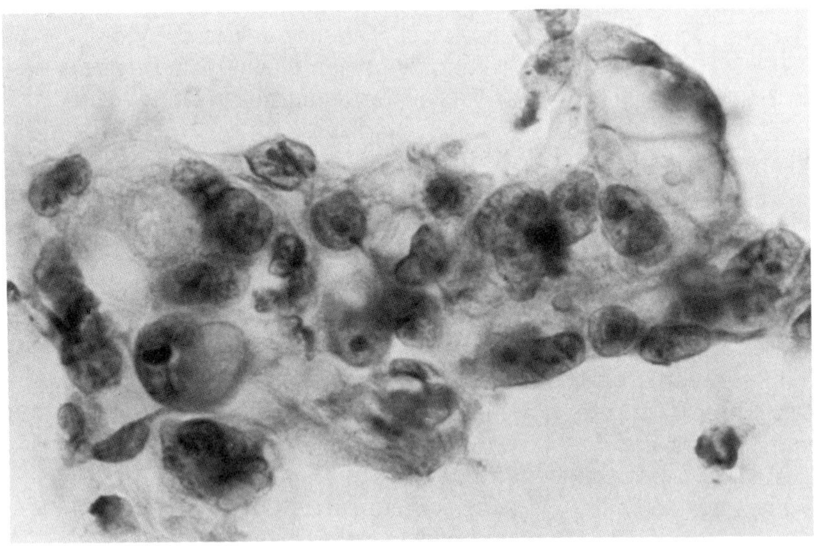

Figure 10-7. Poorly differentiated duct cell adenocarcinoma. A dyshesive cluster of pleomorphic malignant cells with clear or vacuolated cytoplasm and macronucleoli. (Papanicolaou ×400.)

mous cell carcinoma are rare variants of duct cell carcinoma of the pancreas. In the NAB the cancer cells are readily identifiable. Small and large cell anaplastic carcinomas are probably morphologic variants of duct cell carcinoma of the pancreas. In NAB they yield cells similar to those of an oat cell carcinoma or large cell anaplastic carcinoma of the lung.

METASTATIC CANCER

Metastatic carcinomas of the pancreas constitute about 10% of all pancreatic malignant tumors. Among them, cancers originating from the breast, lung, and cutaneous melanomas are the commonest.

AMPULLARY CARCINOMA

The term ampullary carcinoma usually indicates a cancer arising from the ampulla of Vater proper or the intestinal mucosa of the immediate adjacent duodenal mucosa. In advanced cases, the distinction between an ampullary carcinoma and a cancer arising from the pancreatic head or terminal portion of the common bile duct is not possible, and the only diagnosis that can be made in these cases is carcinoma of the ampulla-head-of-pancreas. The majority of these tumors are papillary adenocarcinomas (Fig. 10-8), followed by nonpapillary adenocarcinomas. Adenosquamous carcinoma, mucinous adenocarcinoma, and anaplastic carcinoma of the ampullary region are rare variants, and their cytomorphology is readily identifiable.

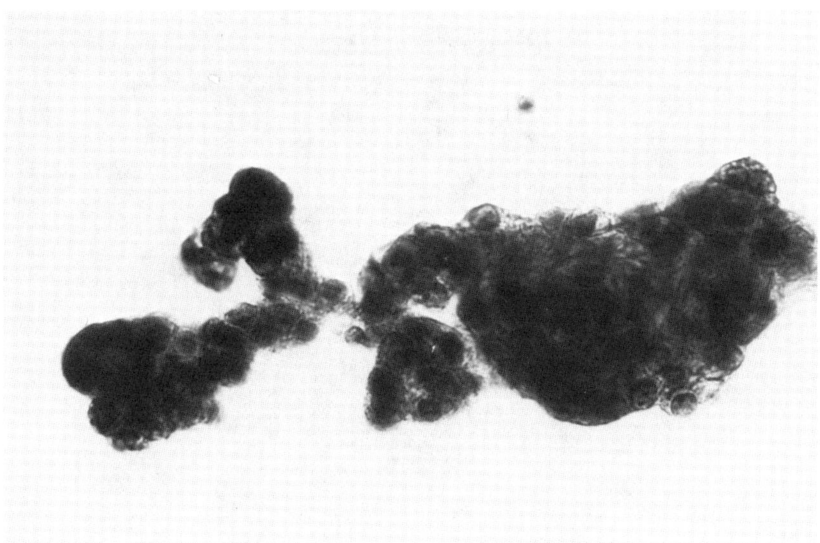

Figure 10-8. Papillary adenocarcinoma of the ampullary region showing a papillary cluster of tumor cells. (Papanicolaou ×250.)

NEUROENDOCRINE TUMOR

These tumors have an unpredictable behavior and may be solitary or multiple. Multiple tumors are usually seen in patients with type I multiple endocrine neoplasia syndrome. They can be nonfunctioning or associated with excessive production of a pancreatic hormone. The tumors vary in size, up to 15 cm or more in diameter. NAB of a pancreatic neuroendocrine tumor reveals fairly regular tumor cells with round nuclei, and ill-defined, sometimes scant, granular cytoplasm. Most commonly, they are seen singly but also they are found in small clusters and rarely in syncytial sheets (Fig. 10-9). Immunocytochemical staining, using antiserum to neuron-specific enolase, shows a strong cytoplasmic reaction. A positive reaction may be expected when antisera to hormones produced by tumor cells (e.g., insulin, glucagon, gastrin, or serotonin) are used. Electron microscopic study of aspirated tumor cells reveals intracytoplasmic clusters of membrane-bound dense-core granules with different features, depending on the types of polypeptide hormone manufactured by the tumor cells.

Distinctive cellular features of duct cell adenocarcinoma, neuroendocrine tumor of the pancreas, and chronic pancreatitis are summarized in Table 10-1.

DIAGNOSTIC ACCURACY

One of the prerequisites for an accurate cytodiagnosis is a cellular and representative sample from the lesion. This depends largely on the skill of the aspirator who does the biopsy on the tumor and on the cytopathologist's experience. For

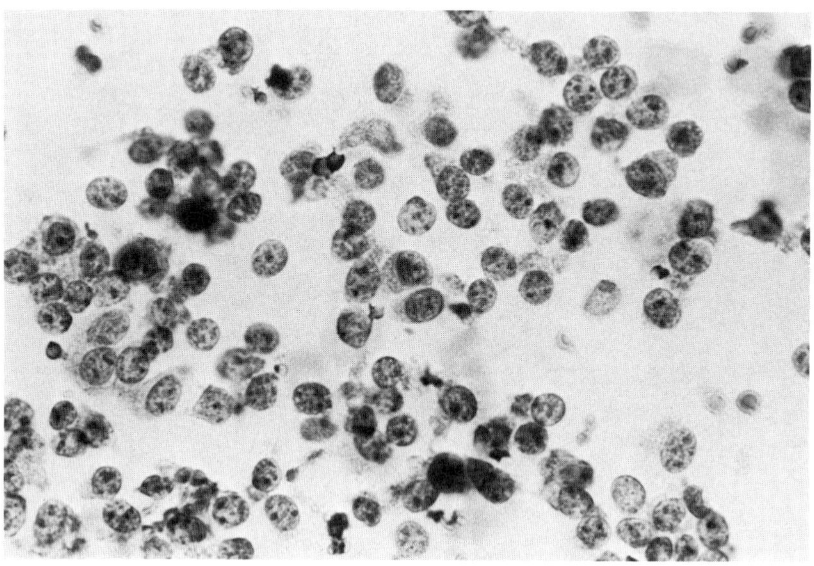

Figure 10-9. Neuroendocrine tumor. Note single and loosely clustered tumor cells with granular ill-defined cytoplasm and round vesicular nuclei showing macronucleoli. (Papanicolaou ×400.)

Table 10-1. Comparative Cytomorphology of Duct Cell Adenocarcinoma, Neuroendocrine Tumor of the Pancreas, and Chronic Pancreatitis

ABC	DUCT CELL ADENOCARCINOMA	NEUROENDOCRINE TUMOR	CHRONIC PANCREATITIS
Cell arrangement	Acini, sheets and singly	Singly and sheets	Sheets and acini
Cell features			
Cytoplasm	Ill-defined	Well- or ill-defined	Well-defined
Nucleus	Oval or pleomorphic Macronucleolus	Round Macronucleolus	Round or oval Nucleolus
Other			
Neuron-specific enolase	−	+	−

peroperative NAB of pancreatic cancers, a diagnostic accuracy of approximately 95% can be anticipated. For percutaneous NAB of pancreatic malignancies, a diagnostic accuracy between 51 and 97% has been reported.

DIAGNOSTIC PITFALLS

False-negative results are mainly due to inadequate or nonrepresentative samples. The false-negative rate of peroperative NAB of pancreatic cancers is about 5% while that of the percutaneous technique varies from 14 to 36%. Other contributing factors to the high false-negative rate of percutaneous NAB of the pancreas include the technique for tumor localization, cystic tumor, and well-differentiation of the neoplasm. Many pancreatic carcinomas are associated with fibrotic chronic pancreatitis and desmoplastic reaction. Thus, they may not yield enough tumor cells for an accurate cytodiagnosis. The fibrotic tumor could also deflect the thin and flexible biopsy needle. Tumor cells aspirated from a well-differentiated adenocarcinoma may display inconspicuous features of malignancy. Multiple biopsies of the tumors often are needed for a positive cytodiagnosis. Aspirate from an area of tumor necrosis may be unsatisfactory for cytologic evaluation, as the tumor cells are not well-preserved. A second biopsy of the thick and peripheral part of the tumor is helpful in this situation. Reactive ductal, acinar, and endothelial cells may have atypical features readily mistaken for cancer cells. Hyperplastic endocrine cells in chronic pancreatitis may display nuclear pleomorphism, mimicking cells of an adenocarcinoma. A careful analysis of the smears often reveals groups of cells with distinct borders and clearly benign-appearing hyperplastic endocrine cells that show only mild atypia.

Aspiration from lesions of the pancreatic head usually samples liver cells which, in a reactive state, often may show large cells with enlarged hyperchromatic nuclei and macronucleoli. Intracytoplasmic yellowish brown bile pigment granules, however, may be observed.

SUGGESTED READING

Al-Kaisi N, Siegler EE: Fine needle aspiration cytology of the pancreas. *Acta Cytol* 1989;33:145–152.

Bell DA: Cytologic features of islet cell tumors. *Acta Cytol* 1987;31:485–492.

Cubilla AL, Fitzgerald PJ: Tumors of the exocrine pancreas. In *Atlas of Tumor Pathology*, series 2. Washington, DC, Armed Forces Institutes of Pathology, 1984.

Fekete PS, Nunez C, Pitlik DA: Fine needle aspiration biopsy of the pancreas: a study of 61 cases. *Diagn Cytopathol* 1986;2:301–306.

Hajdu EO, Kumari-Subaiya S, Phillips G: Ultrasonically guided percutaneous aspiration biopsy of the pancreas. *Semin Diagn Pathol* 1986;3:166–175.

Jones EC, Suen KC, Grant DR, et al.: Fine needle aspiration cytology of neoplastic cysts of the pancreas. *Diagn Cytopathol* 1987;3:238–243.

Kline TS, Goldstein F, Neal HS: Pancreatic carcinoma, pancreatitis and needle aspiration biopsy. *Arch Surg* 1974;109:578–579.

Kline TS: Handbook of aspiration biopsy cytology, ed 2. New York, Churchill Livingstone, 1988, pp 317–341.

Nguyen GK: Percutaneous fine needle aspiration cytology of the pancreas. *Pathol Annu* (Part I) 1985;20:221–238.

Nguyen GK, Rayani NA: Hyperplastic and neoplastic endocrine cells of the pancreas in aspiration biopsy. *Diagn Cytopathol* 1986;2:204–211.

Tao LC, Ho CS, McLaughlin MJ, et al.: Percutaneous fine needle aspiration biopsy of the pancreas. *Acta Cytol* 1978;22:215–220.

11

LIVER, GALLBLADDER, AND BILE DUCTS

Needle aspiration biopsy for cytologic evaluation of tumors and tumor-like lesions of the liver and biliary tree is widely recognized as a safe, suitable, minimally invasive, highly sensitive method for detecting hepatobiliary cancers. The biopsy is usually performed transabdominally, either directly on a palpable tumor or under guidance of a radiologic imaging technique for a nonpalpable mass lesion. Occasionally, it is done on an unsuspected lesion at laparotomy.

INDICATIONS AND CONTRAINDICATIONS FOR NAB

The main indication for NAB of the hepatobiliary tree is to diagnose a primary or a secondary cancer. It may also be used to confirm the benign nature of a space-occupying lesion within the liver. The NAB is contraindicated in patients with bleeding disorders, uncontrolled coughing, or suspected of intraabdominal hydatid cystic disease.

LIVER

Normal Liver

The aspirate from normal liver tissue usually contains numerous hepatocytes, bile duct epithelial cells, and sinusoidal endothelial cells. Kupffer cells are rarely observed. Hepatocytes are round, oval, or polygonal with abundant granular eosinophilic or basophilic cytoplasm. They often occur singly or in small monolayered sheets. The nuclei are central, round, and vesicular and occupy about one-quarter of the cell. The nuclear chromatin is granular and evenly distributed. They show one or two prominent round eosinophilic nucleoli (Fig. 11-1). Mitoses are almost never seen, but polyploid cells are common. Bile duct epithelial cells occur singly or in small clusters of columnar cells that have round, regular, eccentric nuclei. Those from large bile ducts may be found in large sheets showing a honeycomb pattern. The nuclei have a finely granular chromatin pattern and inconspicuous nucleoli (Fig. 11-2). The ducts of Hering are observed, rarely; they are composed of small cuboidal epithelial cells attached to a group of hepatocytes from the end plate. Intercellular bile canaliculi are not seen in smears stained with hematoxylin and eosin or the Papanicolaou technique, but with the amino acid naphthylamidase stain they can be well-visualized as 1.5- to 2-μm bands forming a regular network between hepatocytes. Fragments of sinusoidal or venous endothelium are similar to those of mesothelium. They are composed of polygonal cells with vesicular nuclei containing prominent nucleoli.

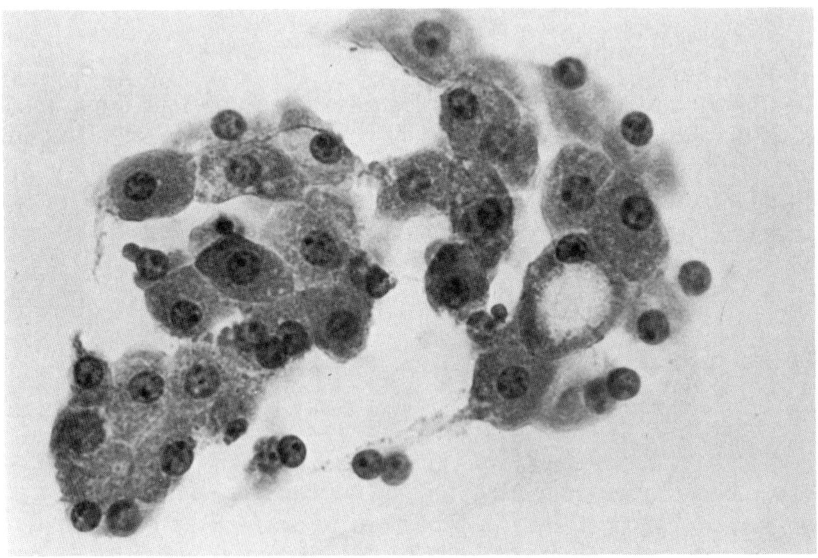

Figure 11-1. Normal liver showing clusters of benign hepatocytes. An abnormal cell with marked fatty changes is also present. (Papanicolaou ×400.)

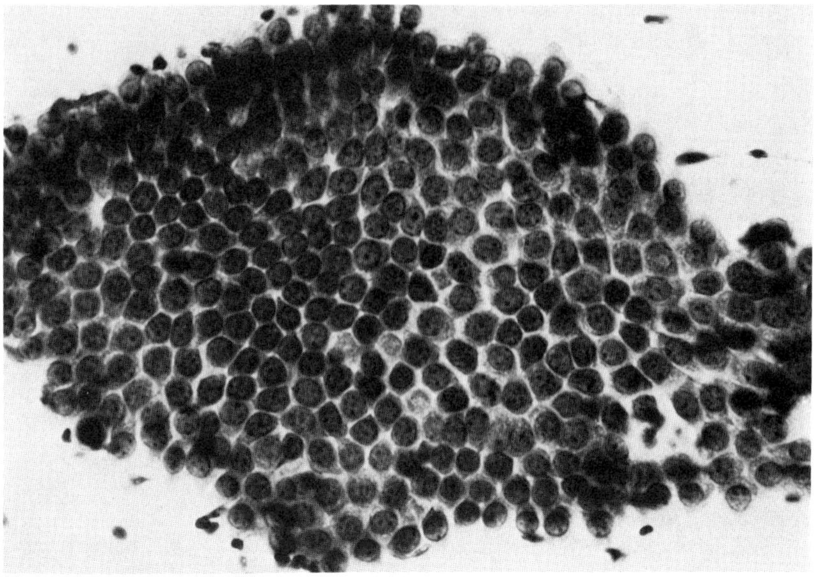

Figure 11-2. A large fragment of bile duct epithelium. (Papanicolaou ×250.)

Benign Hepatic Lesions

Liver abscess. Liver abscesses can be solitary or multifocal. Amebic abscesses are common in tropical countries, but they are exceedingly rare in North America. Needle aspirate from a liver abscess reveals necrotic debris and numerous polymorphonuclear leukocytes. In the case of an amebic abscess, the parasites may be seen in the NAB taken from the abscess wall.

Liver cysts. The solitary or multiple cystic lesions of the liver can be of congenital, parasitic, or neoplastic origins. Most congenital cysts are detected in children but occasionally are found in adults. The NAB from a nonparasitic cyst usually reveals a clear liquid containing a few macrophages and benign columnar or cuboidal epithelial cells. Hydatid cysts of the liver are usually unilocular and located in the right lobe. Cytologic examination of the cyst contents may reveal characteristic hooklets or scoleces with hooklets of the *Echinococcus granulosus* (see Chapter 9, Fig. 9-5).

Focal nodular hyperplasia. The lesion is of unknown pathogenesis. It is usually solitary and is commoner in women than in men. Focal nodular hyperplasia of the liver is usually an incidental finding at laparotomy, but it may be palpable and may lead to surgical resection. Percutaneous NAB yields benign hepatocytes and bile duct epithelial fragments.

Liver cell adenoma. Accumulated data link the development of liver cell adenoma to oral contraceptives, which most of the patients took for more than 5 years.

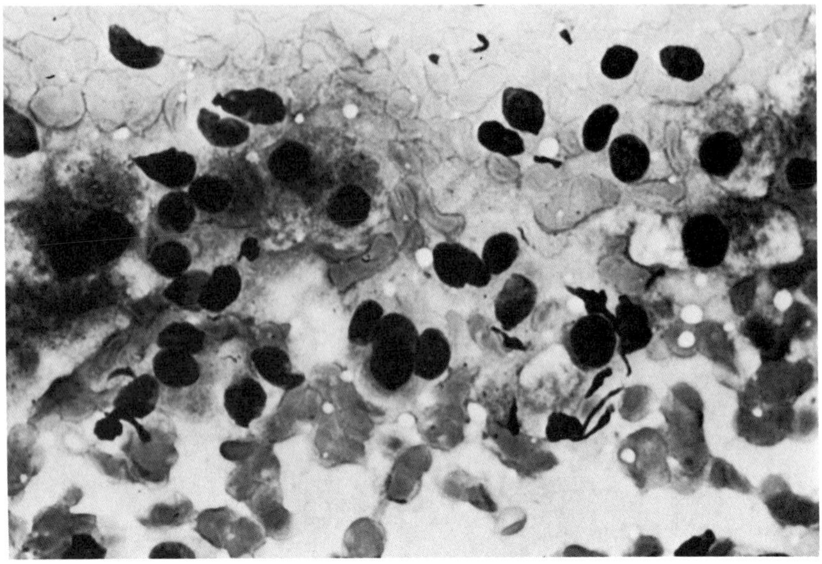

Figure 11-3. Liver cell adenoma showing single and clustered benign-appearing hepatocytes with clear or granular cytoplasm. (Diff-Quik ×400.)

The neoplasms vary from 2 to 30 cm in diameter and may be solitary or multiple. Most are incidentally found at laparotomy, but a high percentage rupture and cause intraabdominal bleeding. NAB reveals benign isolated and clustered liver cells and/or cells similar to hepatocytes with severe fatty change. No bile duct epithelial fragments are noted (Fig. 11-3).

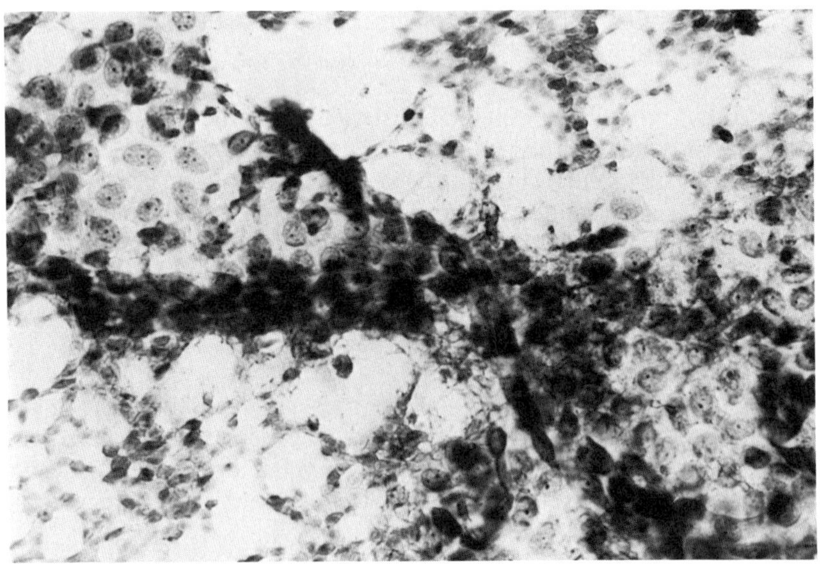

Figure 11-4. Cavernous hemangioma showing a large sheet of endothelial cells. (Papanicolaou ×250.)

Hemangioma. Hepatic hemangiomas are cavernous. They may be solitary or multiple and are variable in size; the lesions may undergo progressive fibrosis with calcification. NAB yields blood and a few irregular sheets of endothelial cells with slight anisokaryosis (Fig. 11-4).

Hepatocellular Carcinoma

Hepatocellular carcinoma occurs worldwide but with great geographic variation in incidence. Although it is a leading cause of death after infancy and childhood in China, Southeast Asia, and most of tropical Africa, it is unusual in Europe and North America. These neoplasms are commonly associated with macronodular cirrhosis, but about 10% arise from a histologically normal liver.

The microscopic appearances of hepatocellular carcinomas are highly diverse, varying from well-differentiated tumors almost indistinguishable from nonneoplastic liver tissue to anaplastic tumors composed of cells barely identifiable as hepatocytes. Cells with clear or vacuolated cytoplasm and pleomorphic or large multinucleated tumor cells may be seen. Bile production, found in a minority of cases, is pathognomonic of this tumor while globular intra- or extracytoplasmic hyaline bodies are present in about 15%. Several histologic patterns have been described, but there is little evidence that any of these morphologic features have biologic or clinical significance. Most are trabecular in their growth; other histologic patterns, e.g., acinar, compact, cirrhous, and papillary, derive from this basic structure. Recently, a special type, the fibrolamellar hepatocellular carcinoma, was identified in young patients. The tumor cells are polygonal with deeply eosinophilic cytoplasm and are surrounded by lamellar fibrosis. This form of neoplasm is usually localized, permitting complete resection and a more favorable prognosis.

Samples obtained by NAB are often hypercellular. The cells display a wide spectrum of morphologic abnormalities, depending on their degree of differentiation.

Well-differentiated tumors with micro- or macrotrabecular patterns yield in NAB benign-appearing hepatocytes with prominent nucleoli. They are seen singly, in variable-sized clusters or in slender or broad fronds, surrounded by or mixed with spindle-shaped endothelial cells (Fig. 11-5).

NAB from a *poorly differentiated neoplasm* reveals isolated and irregularly clustered pleomorphic tumor cells with large nuclei and macronucleoli. Tumor cells showing evidence of bile production, seen as bile plugs within the cell clusters, globular intracytoplasmic inclusions, and fatty changes, may be seen in both well- and poorly differentiated forms. Intranuclear cytoplasmic inclusions are commonly found, but they are not specific, because they can be seen in benign and reactive hepatocytes (Figs. 11-6 – 11-8). Numerous naked tumor cell nuclei are commonly present.

The ABC of *fibrolamellar hepatocellular carcinoma* displays single large tumor cells with abundant, granular, or finely vacuolated, well-demarcated cytoplasm. Large intracytoplasmic pale bodies are commonly seen, and there may be intracytoplasmic globular bodies. The nuclei are usually large and slightly pleomorphic with macronucleoli (Fig. 11-9).

Cellular features of different types of hepatocellular carcinoma are summarized in Table 11-1.

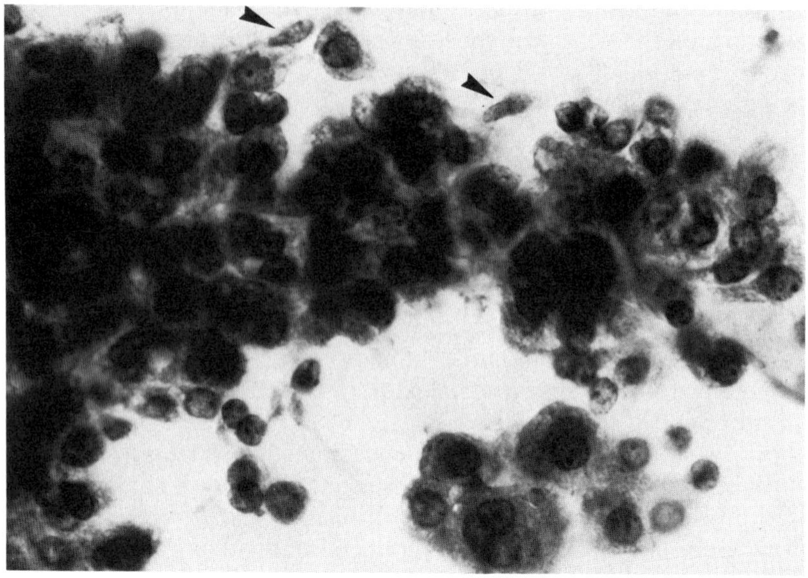

Figure 11-5. Well-differentiated hepatocellular carcinoma. Note broad fronds of benign-appearing hepatocytes mixed with endothelial cells (*arrowhead*). (Papanicolaou ×250.)

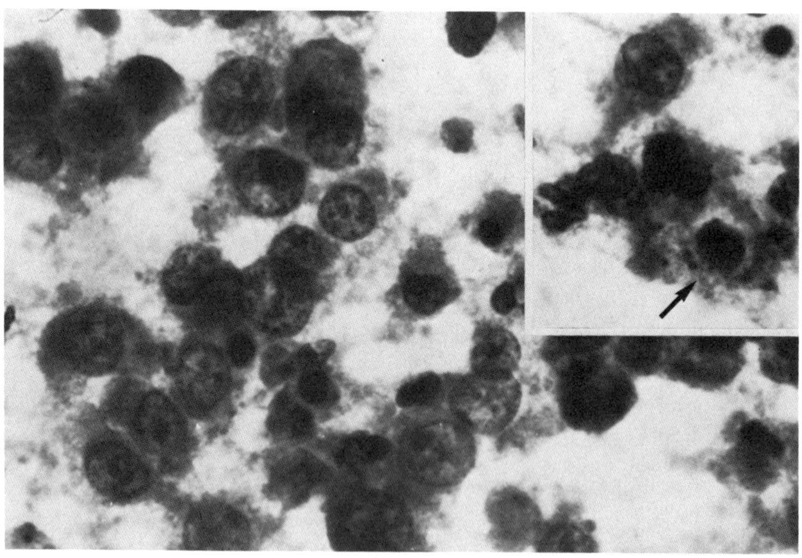

Figure 11-6. Poorly differentiated hepatocellular carcinoma showing pleomorphic malignant cells. **Inset:** A tumor cell containing an eosinophilic intracytoplasmic globular inclusion (*arrow*). (Papanicolaou ×400.)

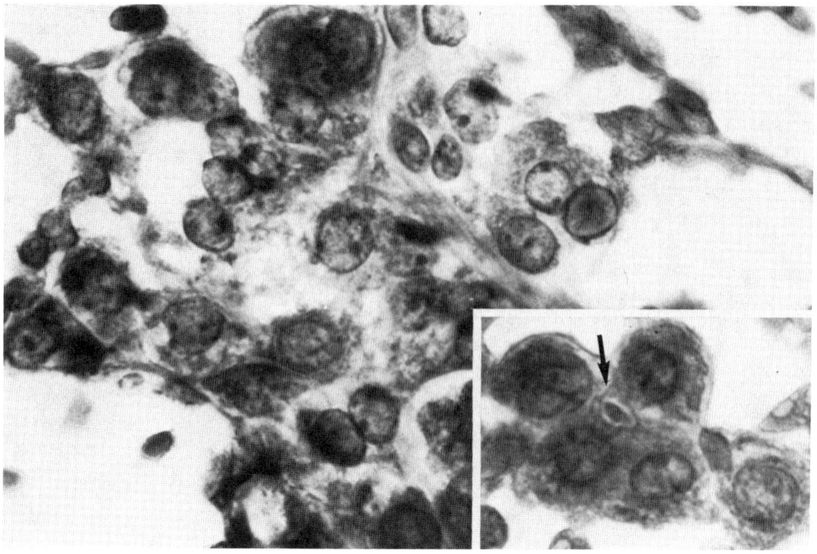

Figure 11-7. Poorly differentiated hepatocellular carcinoma showing dyshesive malignant cells. **Inset:** A group of tumor cells producing bile (*arrow*). (Papanicolaou ×400.)

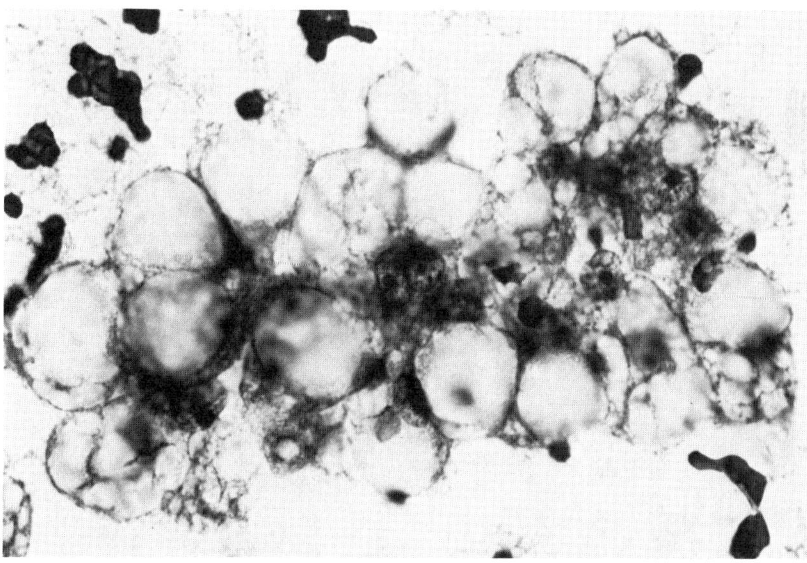

Figure 11-8. Poorly differentiated hepatocellular carcinoma. Note a cluster of tumor cells showing marked fatty changes. (Papanicolaou ×400.)

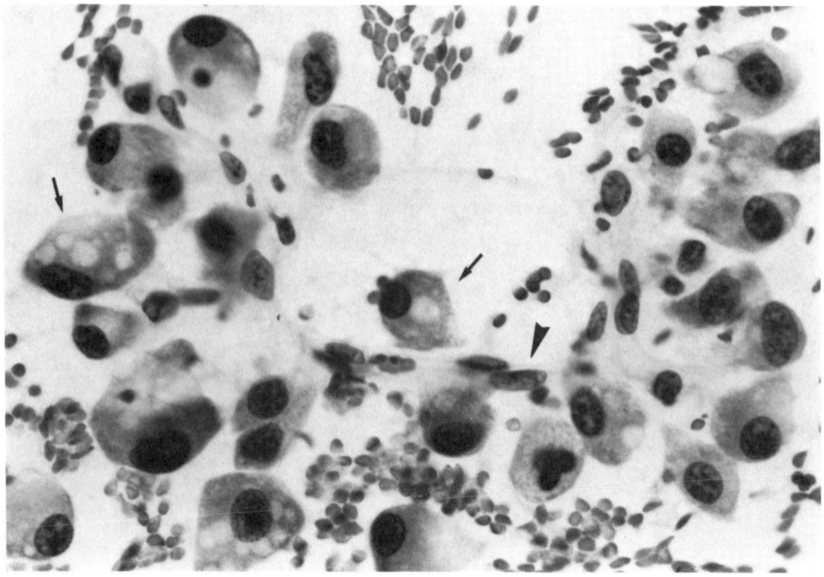

Figure 11-9. Fibrolamellar hepatocellular carcinoma showing isolated large polygonal malignant hepatocytes with granular cytoplasm and intracytoplasmic pale body (*arrow*). A few fibroblasts are present (*arrowhead*). (Papanicolaou ×400.)

Cholangiocarcinoma

Cholangiocarcinoma is an intrahepatic cancer arising from the bile duct epithelium. Although its etiology is unknown, in Eastern countries there is evidence

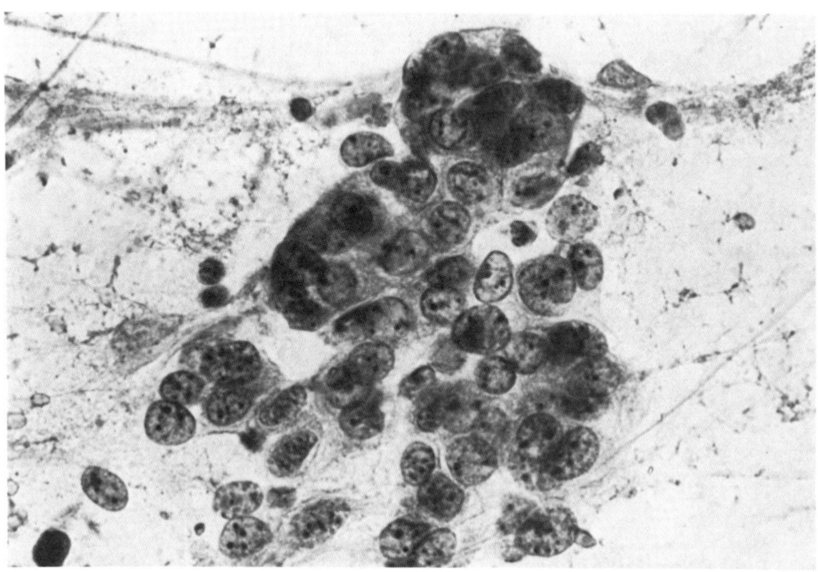

Figure 11-10. Cholangiocarcinoma showing clustered malignant glandular cells. (Papanicolaou ×400.)

Table 11-1. Comparative Cytomorphology of Different Types of Hepatocellular Carcinoma

ABC	WELL-DIFFERENTIATED	POORLY DIFFERENTIATED	FIBROLAMELLAR
Cell arrangement	Papillary fronds, Cohesive clusters with benign endothelial cells	Singly Dyshesive clusters	Singly Dyshesive clusters
Tumor cell[a]			
Shape	Polygonal	Pleomorphic	Polygonal or rounded
Cytoplasm	Well-defined Granular, or vacuolated	Ill-defined Variable	Well-defined Abundant
Cytoplasmic hyaline bodies	+	+++	+
Cytoplasmic pale bodies	+	+	+++

[a] The tumor cells in different types of hepatocellular carcinoma are large and show single or multiple nuclei with single or multiple macronucleoli. Bile production evidenced by bile plugs between two adjacent tumor cells may be seen in all tumors.

suggesting that the tumor is related to the liver flukes. It is usually a solitary adenocarcinoma, although special types occur: mucinous, signet-ring cell, adenosquamous, squamous, and mucoepidermoid carcinomas. Marked desmoplastic reaction is one of its characteristics. There is no way to establish with certainty the identity of a primary bile duct carcinoma on a histologic basis alone, as metastases from carcinomas of the gallbladder, pancreatic ducts, and extrahepatic bile ducts may show similar patterns.

NAB of a cholangioadenocarcinoma reveals clusters of malignant glandular cells (Fig. 11-10).

Metastatic Cancer

Metastatic cancers occur more frequently in the liver than in any other organ and are the most common hepatic neoplasm. Metastatic sarcomas are unusual. Most metastases in the liver arise from abdominal organs drained by the portal vein; primary cancers of the gallbladder, extrahepatic bile ducts, pancreas, and stomach may invade the liver by direct extension. When a patient is known to have cancer, the cytodiagnosis of liver metastasis can be made by comparing the histology or cytology of the primary tumor with the cellular composition of the liver aspirate.

Certain metastatic cancers have fairly specific cytologic features, permitting their identification in ABC with a high degree of accuracy. Among these, bronchogenic oat cell carcinoma, colonic adenocarcinoma, melanoma, neuroendocrine tumor of the pancreas, and renal cell carcinoma generally are readily identifiable (see Chapter 6).

NEOPLASMS OF THE GALLBLADDER AND EXTRAHEPATIC BILE DUCTS

Carcinoma of the gallbladder is more frequent in women and is commonly associated with cholelithiasis. At the time of diagnosis most patients are 50 years of age or older, and the tumor has already invaded the liver. The majority of gallbladder cancers are adenocarcinoma with varying degrees of differentiation. Other rare types of gallbladder cancer are adenosquamous carcinoma, squamous cell carcinoma, undifferentiated carcinoma, carcinoid tumor, melanoma, and lymphoma.

Extrahepatic bile duct carcinoma occurs with equal incidence in men and women in the fifth or sixth decades of life. The tumor may arise at any level of the biliary tree but is more common in the upper third, including the hilum. The majority are well-differentiated mucus-secreting tumors. The NAB reveals groups of malignant glandular cells (Fig. 11-11).

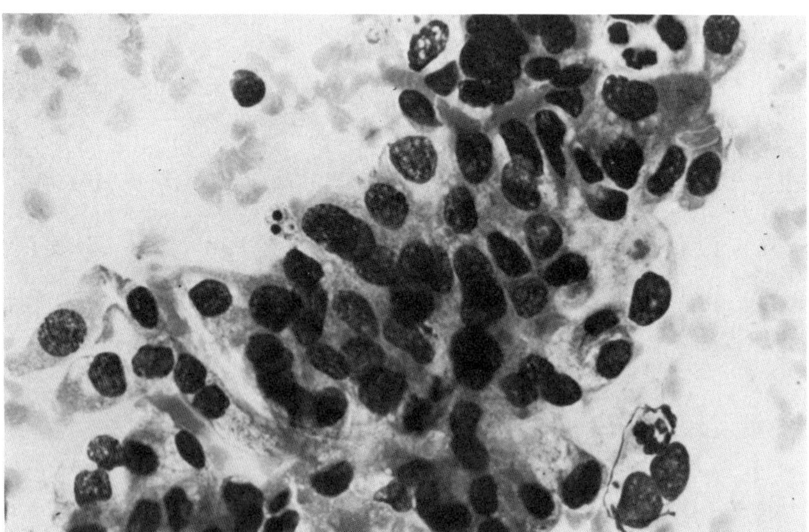

Figure 11-11. Adenocarcinoma of extrahepatic duct showing a fragment of malignant glandular epithelium. (Diff-Quik ×250.)

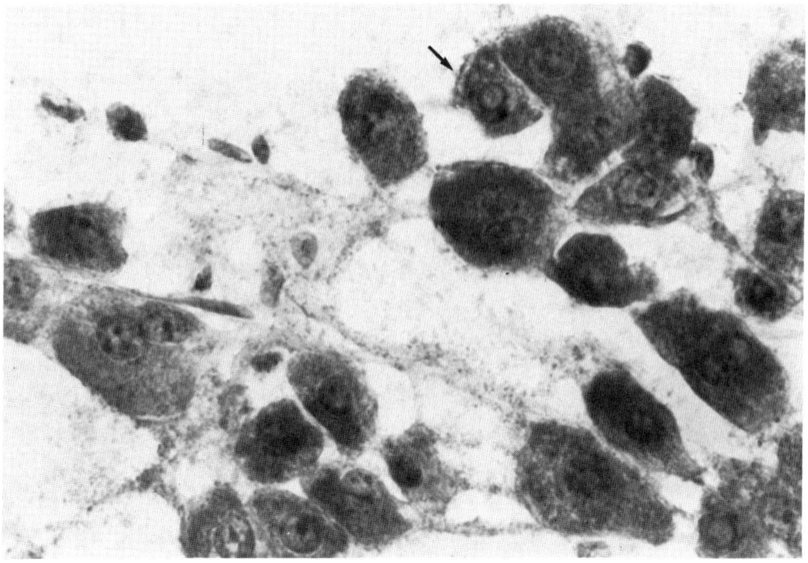

Figure 11-12. Regenerative hepatocytes. Note the large size of the cells and a nucleus showing an intranuclear cytoplasmic inclusion (*arrow*). Several normal-appearing hepatocytes and a few fibroblasts are also present. (Papanicolaou ×400.)

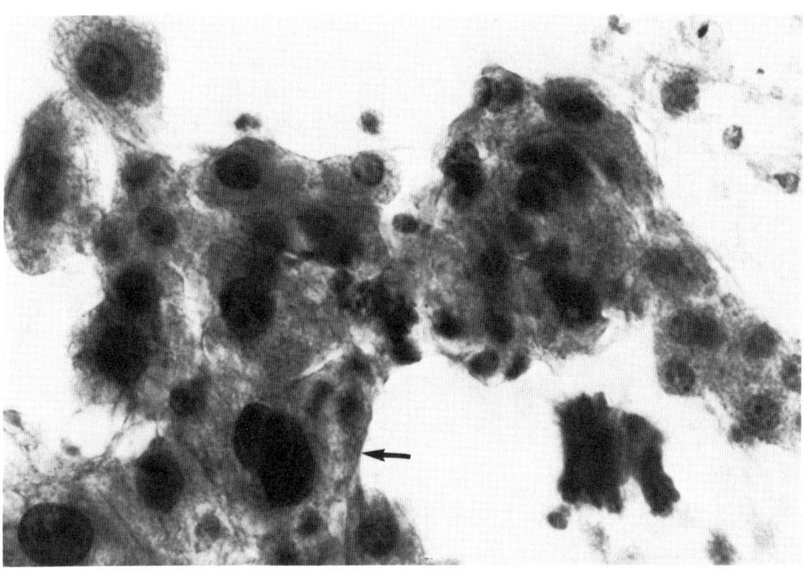

Figure 11-13. Dysplastic hepatocytes showing bizarre and hyperchromatic nuclei (*arrow*) mingled with benign-appearing hepatocytes. (Papanicolaou ×400.)

DIAGNOSTIC ACCURACY AND PITFALLS

Blind liver biopsy with a large-bore needle has a diagnostic sensitivity of 50 to 70% in cases of hepatic cancers, whereas guided NAB has an overall success rate of 70 to 90% (mean, 85%). One of the most important requirements in the cytodiagnosis of liver tumors is a representative sample from the lesion. This largely depends on the skill of the radiologist or clinician performing the biopsy.

There are a few diagnostic pitfalls. These include the identification of regenerative and dysplastic hepatocytes that may mimic malignant liver cells. Regenerative hepatocytes in a liver with metastatic cancer or cirrhosis display large single or multiple nuclei with intranuclear cytoplasmic invaginations. These cells may show marked anisocytosis, but their nuclear chromatin pattern is finely granular (Fig. 11-12). Dysplastic hepatocytes are usually seen in apparently benign liver parenchyma adjacent to a hepatocellular carcinoma or in patients with hepatitis B surface antigen-positive or cirrhosis. They are pleomorphic cells that occur singly and in clusters. Their nuclei are large, containing irregular clumps of chromatin and macronucleoli. When seen in clusters, these malignant-appearing cells are mingled with benign hepatocytes (Fig. 11-13).

SUGGESTED READING

Hidvegi FD: *Guides to Clinical Aspiration Biopsy. Liver and Pancreas*. New York, Igaku-Shoin, 1988.

Nguyen GK: Fine needle aspiration cytology of hepatic tumors in adults. *Pathol Annu* (part I) 1986;22:321–349.

Noguchi S, Yamamoto R, Tatsuta M, et al.: Cell features and patterns in fine needle aspirates of hepatocellular carcinoma. *Cancer* 1986;58:321–328.

Pilotti S, Rilke F, Claren R, et al.: Conclusive diagnosis of hepatic and pancreatic malignancy. *Acta Cytol* 1988;32:27–38.

Rosai J: Liver, gallbladder and extrahepatic bile ducts. In *Ackerman's Surgical Pathology*, ed 7. St. Louis, Mosby, 1989. pp 675–755.

Suen KC: Diagnosis of primary hepatic neoplasms by fine-needle aspiration cytology. *Diagn Cytopathol* 1986;2:99–109.

Tao LC, Kline TS: Liver. In Kline TS: *Handbook of Fine Needle Aspiration Biopsy Cytology, ed* 2. New York, Churchill Livingstone, 1988. pp 343–363.

Wasastejerna C: Liver. In Zajicek J: *Aspiration Biopsy Cytology*, part 2. Basel, S Karger, 1979, pp 167–193.

12

KIDNEY AND ADRENAL

Percutaneous NAB for cytologic evaluation of space-occupying lesions of the kidney and adrenal is a safe and economical diagnostic procedure. It can be accurately performed under the guidance of a radiologic imaging technique. In experienced hands many cases of inflammatory, degenerative, benign, and malignant mass lesions of these organs may be correctly diagnosed, based on cytologic findings, obviating open biopsy for tissue diagnosis. In recent years, the routine use of ultrasonography and computed tomography has detected many clinically silent tumors of the kidney and adrenal in patients investigated for unrelated disorders or during the workup of patients with malignant tumors. NAB of such lesions in cancer patients can provide the oncologist with valuable information about the extent of the disease.

INDICATIONS AND CONTRAINDICATIONS FOR NAB

Any mass lesions of the kidney and adrenal are targets of NAB. The biopsy is contraindicated in patients who have bleeding disorders, bowel distension, or intraabdominal hydatid cysts. Catecholamine-producing adrenal tumors constitute a relative contraindication, since catecholamine "storm" can be pharmacologically prevented.

KIDNEY

Normal Kidney

Normal cells of the kidney may be aspirated during the NAB of a renal mass lesion. The glomeruli appear as multilobulated cellular structures consisting of capillary loops. Cells of proximal convoluted tubules have abundant, ill-defined, granular cytoplasm and round nuclei; they are seen singly or in clusters. Cells of distal convoluted and collecting tubules are smaller than those of proximal convoluted tubules. They are characterized by a well-defined cytoplasm and conspicuous nucleoli. The loops of Henle are thin tubules consisting of cuboidal cells with scant cytoplasm and ovoid nuclei (Fig. 12-1). The NAB from the renal pelvis reveals droplets of urine containing a few benign urothelial cells with well-defined cytoplasm and round nuclei.

Benign Renal Mass Lesions

Solitary benign renal cysts are found in about 50% of people over the age of 55. They are clinically silent and may be large. NAB of these lesions yields clear yellow fluid containing a few benign cuboidal epithelial lining cells and foam cells. If the cyst content is hemorrhagic, a renal cancer with necrotic degenerative changes should be suspected. Because some cystic renal cell carcinomas have a clear fluid content, however, all cyst contents should be examined cytologically to rule out the possibility of a carcinoma.

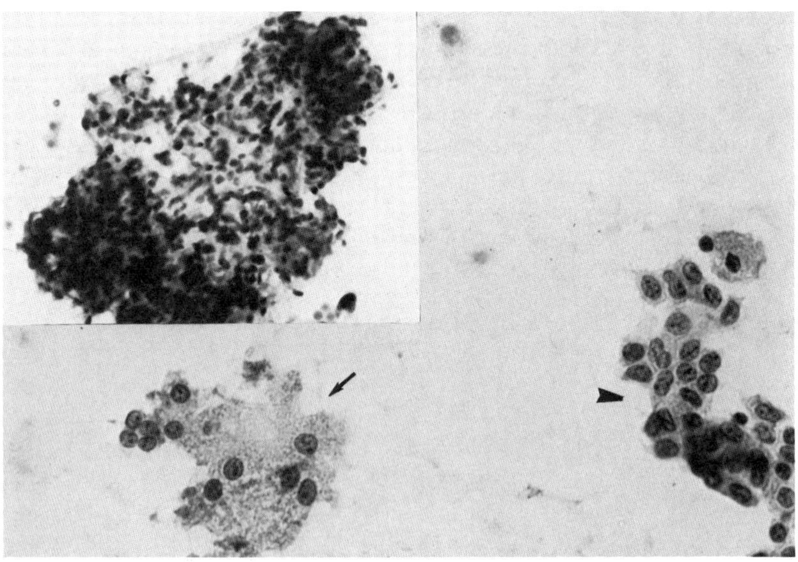

Figure 12-1. Cytology of the normal kidney showing a group of proximal convoluted tubule cells (*arrow*) and a fragment of distal convoluted tubule epithelium (*arrowhead*). **Inset:** A vascular glomerulus. (Hematoxylin and eosin ×250; **Inset** ×100).

Renal angiomyolipoma is a benign tumor consisting of an intimate mixture of mature fatty tissue, smooth muscle cells, and blood vessels in different proportions. The smooth muscle cells may display bizarre morphology. This tumor may occur as multiple and bilateral lesions in 50 to 80% of patients with tuberosclerosis or as a solitary lesion in patients with no clinical evidence of tuberosclerosis. In the latter situation the distinction between this lesion and a renal cell carcinoma is challeng-

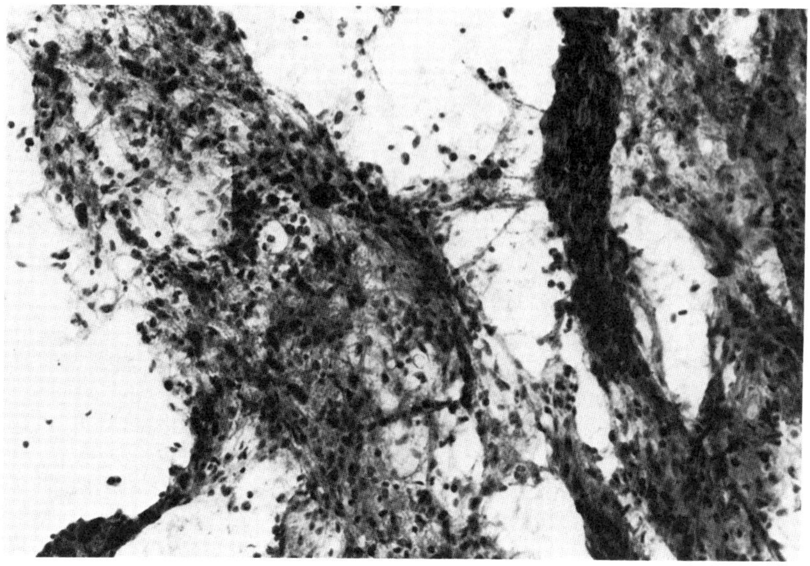

A

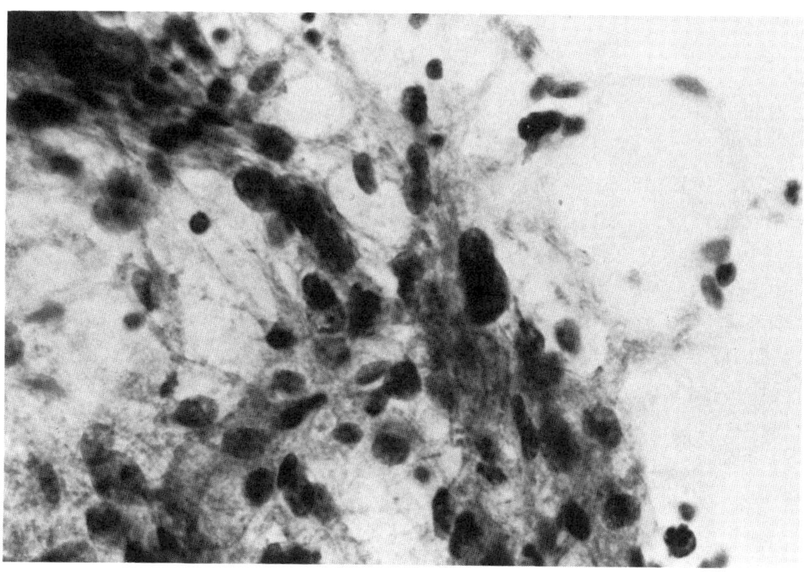

B

Figure 12-2. Renal angiomyolipoma. **A.** Clusters of benign smooth muscle cells mixed with mature fat cells. **B.** Bundles of smooth muscle cells showing bizarre nuclei. (Papanicolaou. **A** ×100, **B** ×400.)

ing. ABC of the lesion reveals sheets of endothelial cells, clusters of smooth muscle cells, and groups of mature fat cells (Fig. 12-2A). Atypical smooth muscle cells may be seen (Fig. 12-2B).

Renal oncocytoma is an uncommon lesion that can be solitary or multiple. Although its diagnosis may be suggested by preoperative NAB, however, its correct diagnosis requires an extensive microscopic examination of the resected tumor. When a renal oncocytoma is suspected, the tumor should be removed by partial nephrectomy, if technically feasible, and examined by frozen section for possible renal cell carcinoma. NAB of a renal oncocytoma may show numerous polygonal cells, singly or in loose clusters. The tumor cells have abundant, granular, well-defined cytoplasm and small round nuclei showing inconspicuous nucleoli (Fig. 12-3).

Malignant Renal Tumors

Renal cell carcinoma has peak incidence in the fifth and sixth decades of life and constitutes less than 3% of all cancers in adults. Histologically, it is composed of clear or granular cells arranged in acinar, solid, or papillary patterns. Rarely, it is focally or completely sarcomatoid. Based on nuclear features, it may be classified into three grades. Grade 1 tumors are characterized by cells having small and regular nuclei with inconspicuous nucleoli. In grade 2 tumors, the cells have regular but larger nuclei with prominent nucleoli. Grade 3 tumors consist of bizarre and/or sarcomatoid cells showing large pleomorphic nuclei with irregular macronucleoli. Multiple grades may coexist in about 15% of the tumors.

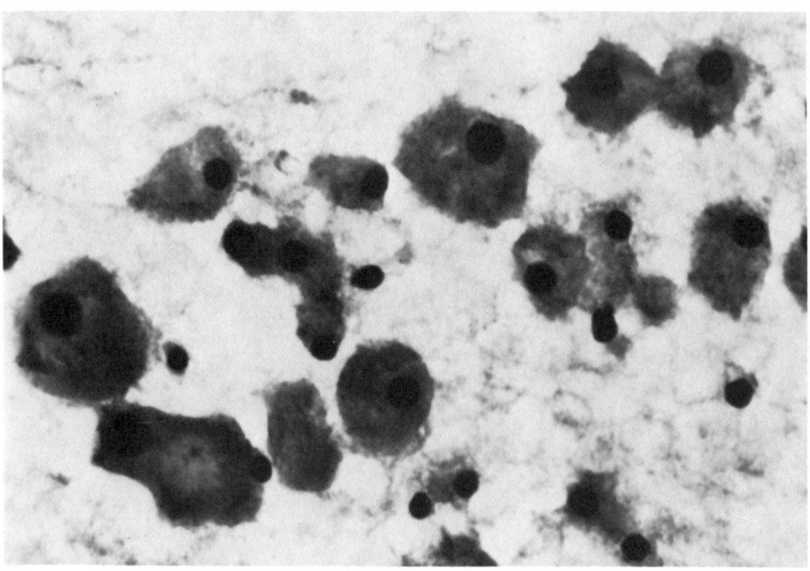

Figure 12-3. Renal oncocytoma. Single and clustered polygonal oncocytic tumor cells. (Papanicolaou ×400.)

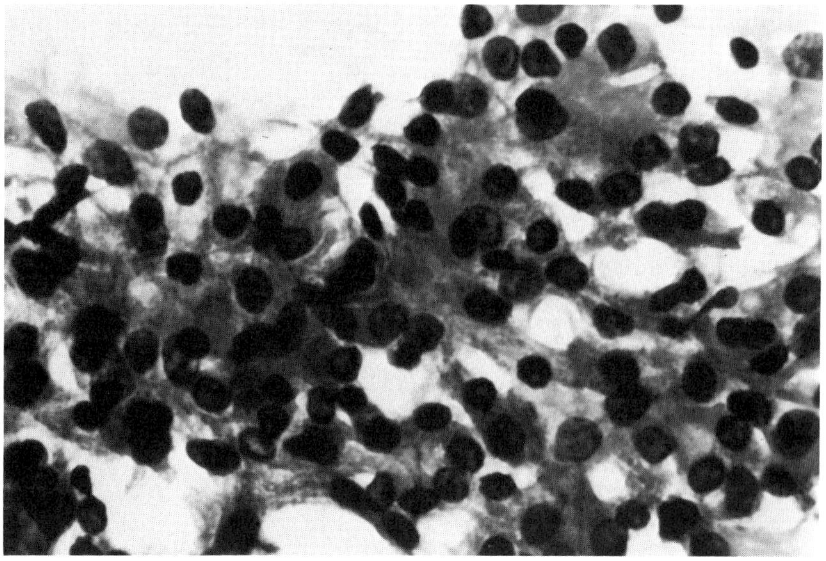

Figure 12-4. Renal cell carcinoma grade 1. A large sheet of tumor cells showing small nuclei and granular or clear cytoplasm. (Papanicolaou ×400.)

Aspirates from renal cell carcinomas are cellular and usually show cohesive and large clusters of tumor cells and necrotic debris (Figs. 12-4 and 12-5). Single and small groups of tumor cells may also be present. Naked tumor cell nuclei are commonly observed. Foamy histiocytes are seen in aspirates from the papillary

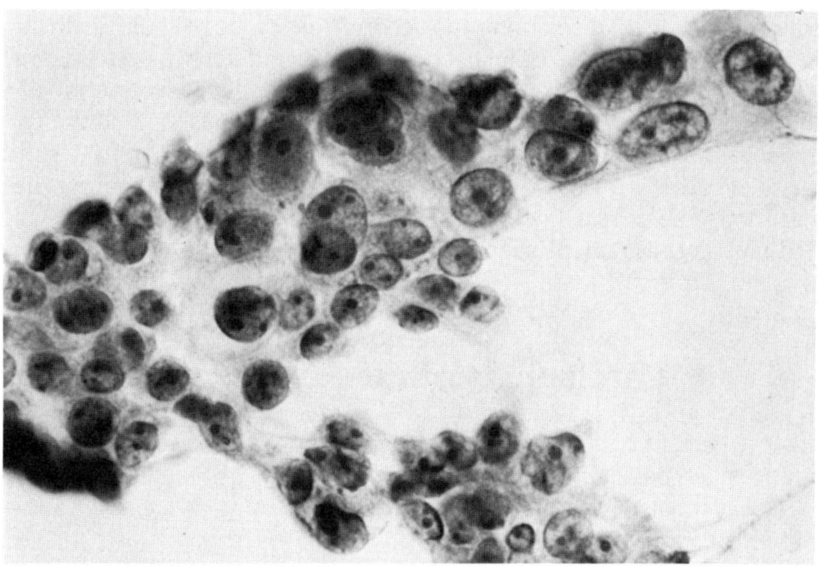

Figure 12-5. Renal cell carcinoma grade 3 showing a dyshesive sheet of tumor cells with indistinct cytoplasmic borders and with macronucleoli. (Papanicolaou ×400.)

Table 12-1. Comparative Cytomorphology of Renal Oncocytoma and Renal Cell Carcinoma

ABC	ONCOCYTOMA	CARCINOMA GRADE 1	CARCINOMA GRADE 2	CARCINOMA GRADE 3
Cell arrangement	Single	Large sheets Dyshesive cells	Large sheets Dyshesive cells	Smaller sheets Dyshesive cells
Tumor cells				
Configuration	Polygonal	Polygonal	Polygonal	Pleomorphic
Cytoplasm	Abundant and granular	Abundant, clear or granular	Abundant, clear or granular	Variable, clear or granular
Nuclei	Small, round	Small, oval	Larger, oval	Pleomorphic
Nucleoli	Inconspicuous	Small or conspicuous	Macronucleoli	Macronucleoli
Naked nuclei	−	±	++	+++

type. Table 12-1 summarizes distinctive cytologic findings of renal oncocytoma and carcinoma.

Wilms' tumor, or nephroblastoma, is the commonest renal cancer in children, reaching its peak incidence during the second year of life. Histologically, a classic nephroblastoma has three cellular components: undifferentiated blastematous, epithelial, and stromal elements. The tumor stroma varies considerably in composition and structure and may show muscle, fat, cartilaginous, and neural cells. The epithelial elements may form tubular structures consisting of basaloid, squamous, or glandular cells. NAB from a classic Wilms tumor reveals blastematous elements, spindle-shaped cells, and sheets or clusters of epithelial cells (Fig. 12-6). Smooth or striated muscle cells may be seen.

Carcinomas of the Renal Pelvis

Ninety percent of all renal pelvic tumors are transitional cell carcinomas, and 85% of them are papillary in configuration. Squamous cell carcinomas account for only 7% of all renal pelvic cancers, whereas undifferentiated carcinoma and adenocarcinoma are very rare.

Depending on the degree of cellular atypia, transitional cell carcinomas of the renal pelvis may be divided into three grades. NAB of a grade 1 tumor shows large clusters of urothelial cells with minimal nuclear atypia which, in conjunction with a space-occupying lesion demonstrated by pyelography, are suggestive of the tumor

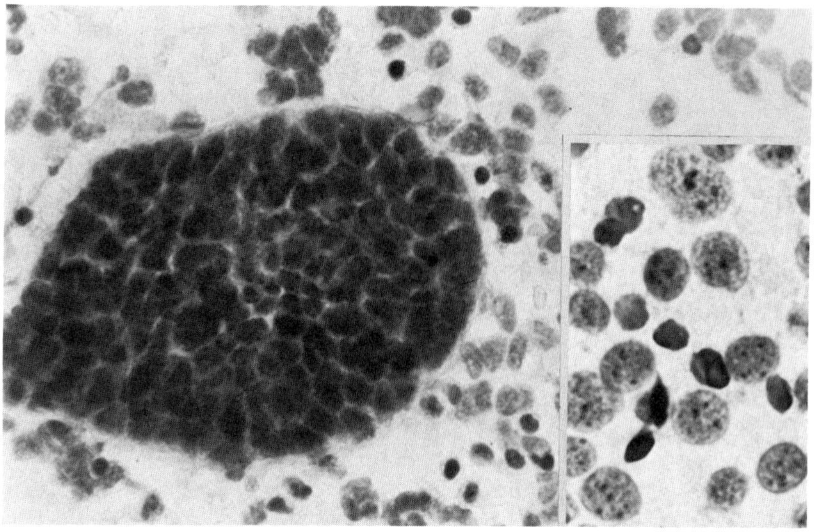

Figure 12-6. Wilms tumor. A cohesive fragment of tumor epithelium with basaloid cells and single round blastematous elements. **Inset:** Blastematous cell at higher magnifications. (Papanicolaou ×250; **Inset** ×400.)

(Fig. 12-7). Higher-grade tumors will yield malignant urothelial cells singly or in clusters (Fig. 12-8).

Squamous cell carcinoma, adenocarcinoma, and undifferentiated carcinoma, respectively, will show in NAB malignant squamous, glandular, and anaplastic cells in clusters or singly.

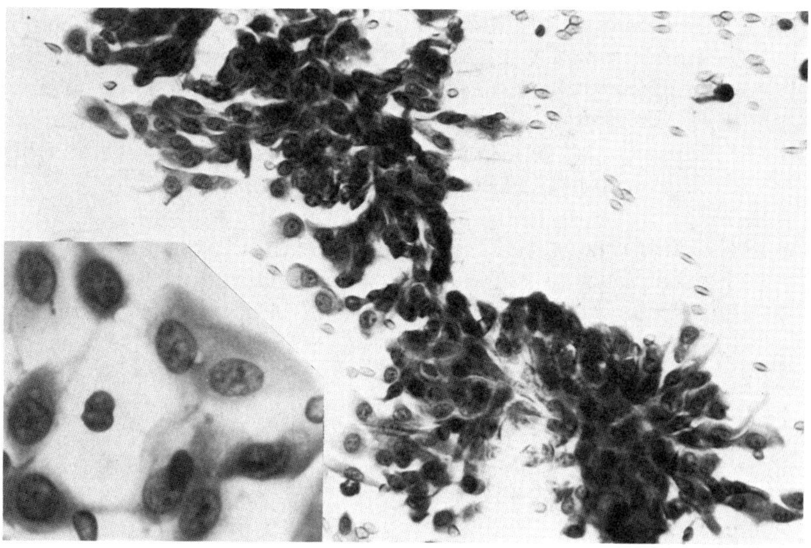

Figure 12-7. Papillary transitional cell carcinoma grade 1 showing large papilla-like clusters of tumor cells with minimal nuclear atypia. (Papanicolaou ×100; **Inset** ×400.)

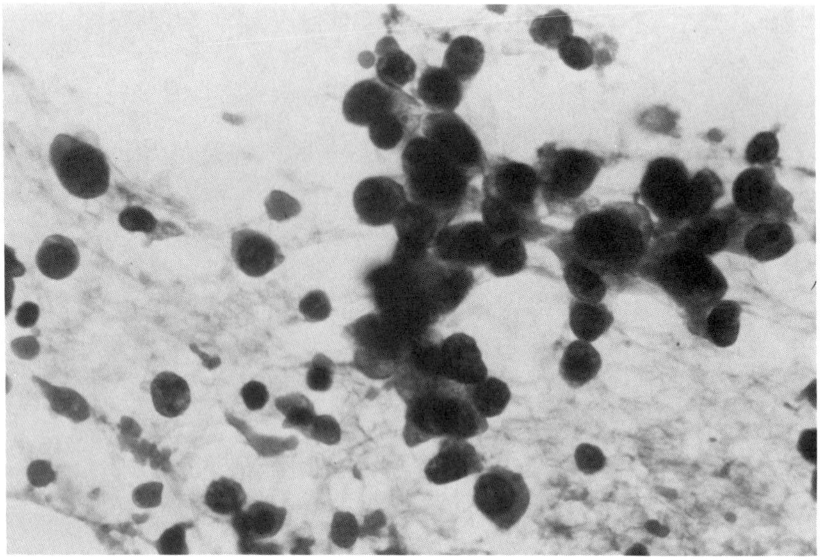

Figure 12-8. Papillary transitional cell carcinoma grade 2 showing single and dyshesive groups of malignant urothelial cells with ill-defined cytoplasm and high nuclear cytoplasmic ratio. (Papanicolaou ×400.)

ADRENAL

Tumors of the Cortex

Adrenal cortical adenoma is often a solitary, well-encapsulated, nonfunctioning tumor that is generally an incidental finding during investigation of an unrelated problem. The tumor is usually smaller than 5 cm in greatest dimension and consists of cells with morphologic features similar to those of the zona fasciculata or zona glomerulosa of the normal adrenal cortex. The NAB reveals numerous naked, round, and regular nuclei and large polygonal cells with vacuolated cytoplasm. Occasionally, cells with nuclear atypias may be present (Fig. 12-9).

Adrenal cortical carcinomas can occur at any age and may be clinically nonfunctioning or associated with a number of clinical manifestations such as aldosteronism, Cushing's syndrome, and polycythemia. The tumor is usually large when it is discovered. Histologically, there are a wide range of microscopic patterns consisting of benign-appearing cells resembling those of the normal adrenal cortex or anaplastic cancer cells. Two important criteria of malignancy are numerous mitoses and vascular invasion. The NAB may show benign-appearing polygonal epithelial cells present singly, in clusters, or in large sheets (Fig. 12-10). In other cases, single and clustered bizarre cancer cells are seen.

Tumors of the Medulla

Pheochromocytoma arises from paraganglionic cells and may occur at any age. About 10% of pheochromocytomas are located outside of the adrenal. The tumor

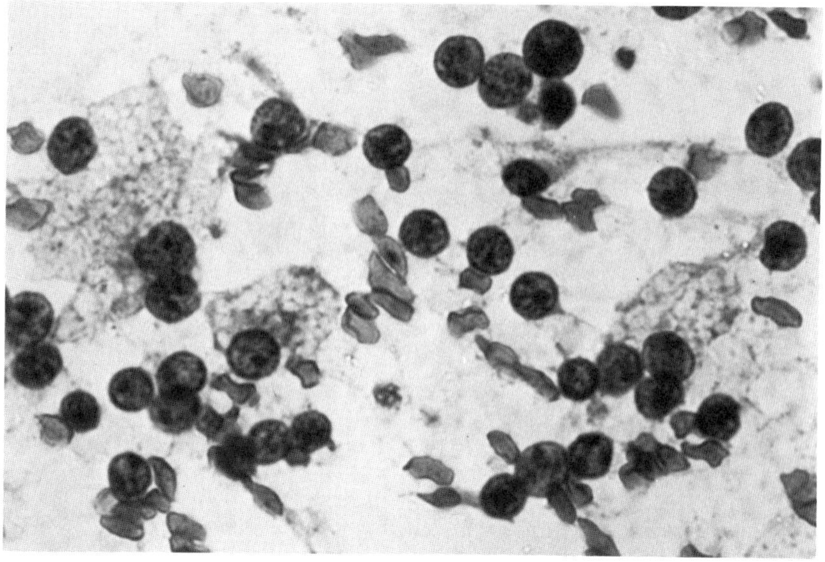

Figure 12-9. Adrenal cortical adenoma. Numerous naked round nuclei and a few polygonal cell with foamy or vacuolated cytoplasm. (Papanicolaou ×400.)

may be functional or nonfunctional, depending on its ability to produce enough catecholamines to cause signs and symptoms. Histologically, pheochromocytoma is characterized by nests of polygonal or fusiform tumor cells separated by fibrovascular septae. The tumor cells usually show pleomorphic nuclei, prominent nucleoli, and granular cytoplasm containing argyrophilic granules. The NAB reveals numerous single and clustered tumor cells, showing ill-defined granular cytoplasm and

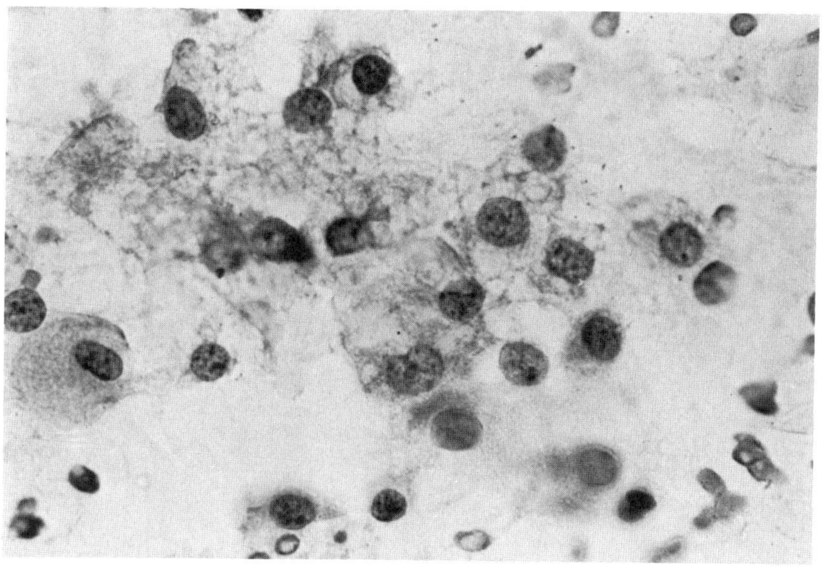

Figure 12-10. Adrenal cortical carcinoma. A sheet of tumor cells with clear and vacuolated cytoplasm. (Papanicolaou ×400.)

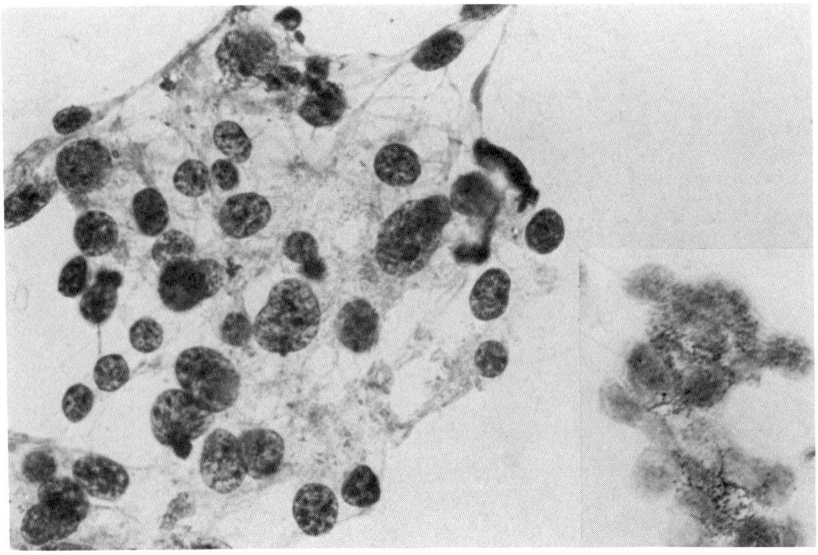

Figure 12-11. Pheochromocytoma. Sheets of bizarre cells with ill-defined cytoplasm and pleomorphic nuclei. **Inset:** Intracytoplasmic argyrophil brown black granules. (Papanicolaou ×400; **Inset:** Grimelius staining ×400.)

round or oval nuclei with irregular chromatin pattern (Fig. 12-11). Their cytoplasm shows brown-black granules with argyrophil staining and reacts positively with neuron-specific enolase antiserum. Intracytoplasmic neurosecretory-type granules may be demonstrated by an electron microscopic study of aspirated tumor cells.

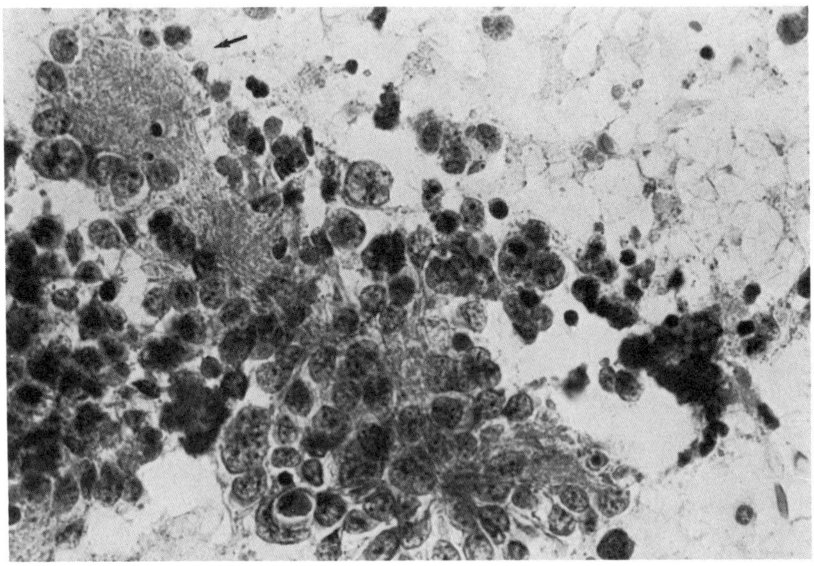

Figure 12-12. Ganglioneuroblastoma showing single and clustered round malignant cells and an immature ganglion cell (arrow) (Papanicolaou ×400.)

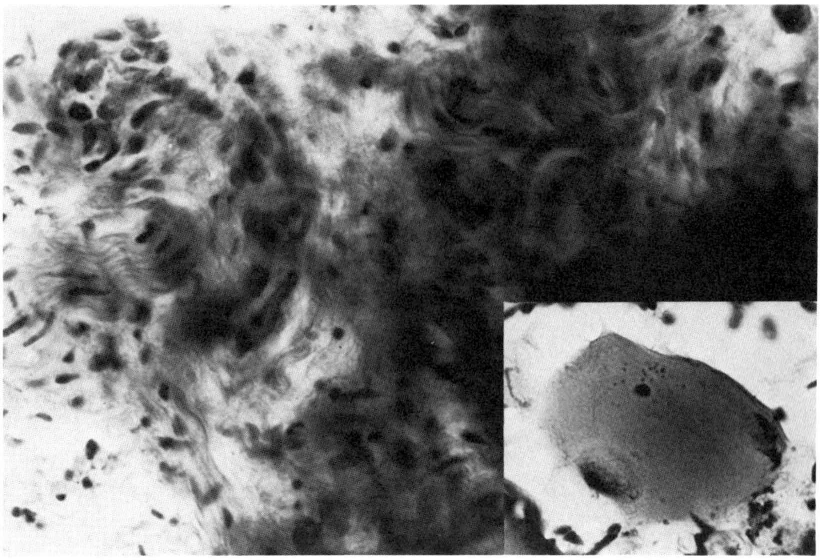

Figure 12-13. Ganglioneuroma showing tight bundles of nerve fibers with spindle-shaped nuclei. **Inset:** A mature ganglion cell. (Papanicolaou ×250, **Inset** ×400.)

Neuroblastoma, ganglioneuroblastoma, and ***ganglioneuroma*** represent different stages of maturation of tumors arising from the sympathetic nervous system. Neuroblastoma is the most immature neoplasm of the group. It is almost always unilateral, and most cases are detected in children under 4 years of age. Histologically, neuroblastoma is composed of small malignant cells with scant cytoplasm forming rosettes around central areas filled with filamentous and granular material. NAB from the tumor yields numerous malignant small cells with round hyperchromatic nuclei, and ill-defined cytoplasm present singly or in groups forming rosettes. The ABC of ganglioneuroblastoma shows, in addition to neuroblasts, several multinucleated ganglion cells (Fig. 12-12). Ganglioneuroma is the fully differentiated member of the group. It usually shows in NAB scanty cellular material containing a few bundles of nerve fibers, naked carrot-shaped nuclei, and mature ganglion cells (Fig. 12-13).

Cellular features of tumors of the adrenal are summarized in Table 12-2.

Metastatic Cancer

The adrenal is a common site of metastases of cancers arising from other organs. Of these cancers, bronchogenic carcinomas are the most frequent, followed by carcinomas of the breast, stomach, colon, pancreas, and kidney, and then cutaneous melanoma. The cytodiagnosis of metastatic cancers to the adrenals usually can be established by comparison of the ABC with cytologic or histologic materials from the known primary tumor. It should be borne in mind that about 50% of all adrenal masses found in cancer patients are benign.

Table 12-2 Cytomorphology of Adrenal Tumors

ABC	CORTICAL ADENOMA	CORTICAL CARCINOMA	PHEOCHROMOCYTOMA	NEUROBLASTOMA
Cell arrangement	Singly or loose clusters	Singly or dyshesive clusters	Dyshesive clusters	Singly or rosettes containing granular or fibrillary material
Tumor cells				
Configuration	Polygonal	Polygonal or slightly pleomorphic	Pleomorphic	Round and regular
Cytoplasm	Well-defined; clear or vacuolated	Well- or ill-defined; clear, vacuolated or granular	Ill-defined, granular	Ill-defined, fibrillary
Nuclei	Round Nucleoli	Round Macronucleoli	Oval, or pleomorphic Macronucleoli	Round Macronucleoli
Naked nuclei	+++	+++	+	+
Other				
Neuron-specific enolase	–	–	+	+
Grimelius-positive granules	–	–	+	+

DIAGNOSTIC ACCURACY AND PITFALLS

In experienced hands the success rate of cytodiagnosis of tumors of the kidney and adrenal is high: over 90% for both sites.

The cytodiagnosis of tumors of the kidney and adrenal is usually not problematic. However, diagnostic difficulties may be encountered in cases with inadequate cell samples. Not only do the cells of a renal oncocytoma mimic normal hepatocytes but also liver cells in ABC of a tumor arising from the upper pole of the right kidney may be a contaminant. Samples from a renal oncocytoma should also be screened carefully for cohesive clusters and sheets of cells with clear cytoplasm characteristic of well-differentiated renal cell carcinoma, because some renal cell carcinomas have focal oncocytic features. Another source of error is the presence of bizarre smooth muscle cells in ABC of a renal angiomyolipoma; a careful search should be made for irregular clusters of benign fatty tissue mixed with benign smooth muscle cells. Blastematous cells of a Wilms tumor may mimic cells of a lymphoma, neuroblastoma, or an extrarenal sarcoma invading the kidney. Immunocytochemical staining using leukocyte common antigen, S-100 protein and vimentin antisera are helpful in this situation. The differential diagnosis between an adrenal cortical carcinoma and a renal cell carcinoma invading or metastatic to the adrenal is a well-known difficulty histologically and cytologically. Immunocytochemical studies are not helpful in this situation, as cells of both tumors usually express vimentin and keratin, as well as other epithelial antigens. By electron microscopy, cells of the latter may show numerous smooth endoplasmic reticula while those of the former show microvilli, abundant glycogen granules, fat droplets, and mitochondria, as well as rough endoplasmic reticula.

SUGGESTED READING

Analen KA, Tyrkko JES, Nurmi MJ: Aspiration biopsy cytology of renal oncocytoma. *Acta Cytol* 1985;29:859–862.

Katz RL, Patel S, MacKay B, et al.: Fine needle aspiration cytology of the adrenal. *Acta Cytol* 1984;28:269–282.

Koss LG, Woyke S, Olszewski W: *Aspiration Biopsy. Cytologic Interpretation and Histologic Bases*. New York, Igaku-Shoin, 1984. pp 394–421.

Murphy WM, Zambroni BR, Emerson LD, et al.: Aspiration biopsy of the kidney. Simultaneous collection of cytologic and histologic specimens. *Cancer* 1985;26:200–205.

Nguyen GK: Percutaneous fine needle aspiration biopsy cytology of the kidney and adrenal. *Pathol Annu* 1987;21(1):163–191.

Nurmi M, Tyrkko J, Puntala P, et al.: Reliability of aspiration biopsy cytology in the grading of renal adenocarcinoma. *Scand J Urol Nephrol* et al.: 1984;18:151–156.

Plotti S, Rilke, F, Alasio L, et al.: The role of fine needle aspiration in the assessment of renal masses. *Acta Cytol* 1988;32:1–10.

Suen KC: *Guides to Clinical Aspiration Biopsy. Retroperitoneum and Intestine*. New York, Igaku-Shoin, 1987. pp 131–189.

Tao LC: *Transabdominal Fine Needle Aspiration Biopsy. New York, Igaku-Shoin*, 1990. pp 179–284.

13

CENTRAL NERVOUS SYSTEM

CT-guided stereotactic needle biopsy of a brain tumor performed under local anesthesia through a burr hole in the skull now is a routine diagnostic procedure in many hospitals with neurosurgery services. However, the small size of the specimens procured by the biopsy needle makes their pathologic examination by frozen sections difficult. Use of crush preparations of brain tissue as a supplement to frozen sections for the rapid intraoperative diagnosis of specimens that are usually sampled by a 14- to 22-gauge needle with or without a core device or a cup forceps has proved to be a valuable technique. Smears are usually prepared from tiny tissue fragments that are unsuitable for frozen sections. They are stained with hematoxylin and eosin.

INDICATIONS AND CONTRAINDICATIONS FOR NAB

CT-guided stereotactic needle biopsy is the preferred diagnostic procedure in handling patients who are poor operative candidates and those with deeply situated brain tumors that are inaccessible to open biopsy. It provides morphologic evidence of unresectable brain cancers that can be treated with radiation and chemotherapeutic agents. It permits easily obtainable periodic biopsies to detect possible recurrences of gliomas, and it is also helpful in investigating nonneoplastic space-occupying lesions and radiation-induced necrosis of the brain that may mimic a mass lesion on CT scanning. The technique may also be used for spatial delimitations of gliomas. It is contraindicated in patients with bleeding diathesis.

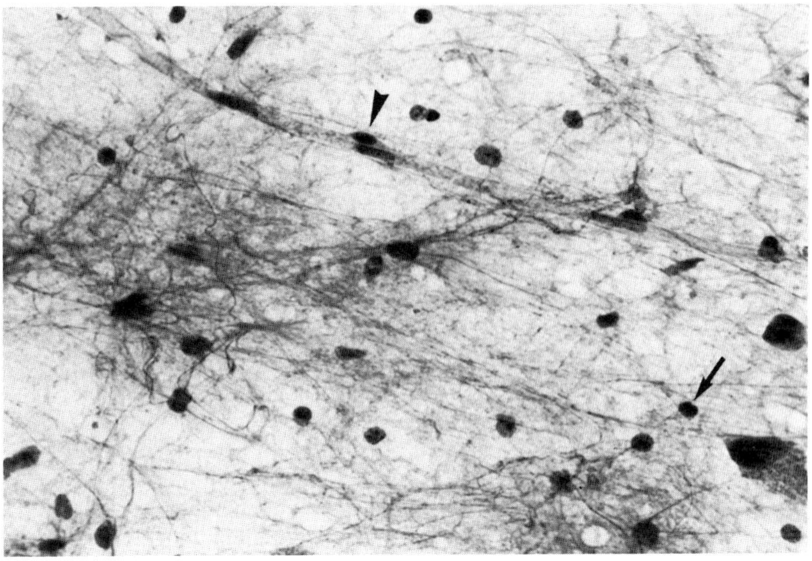

Figure 13-1. Normal brain. Note the small hyperchromatic nuclei of oligodendrocytes (*arrow*) and larger vesicular nuclei of astrocytes and fragments of capillary vessel (*arrowhead*). A neuron with granular cytoplasm and large nucleus with prominent nucleolus is seen at the *lower right corner* of the figure. (Hematoxylin and eosin ×250.)

NORMAL CEREBRUM

Crush preparation of normal cerebral tissue reveals numerous benign glial cells located in a fibrillary background containing capillary vessels. The spider-like cytoplasmic extensions of astrocytes and their vesicular nuclei can be well-visualized. Oligodendrocytes show smaller and hyperchromatic nuclei. Triangular-shaped neurons are larger cells and show granular cytoplasm and large vesicular nuclei with macronucleoli (Fig. 13-1).

REACTIVE GLIOSIS

Reactive gliosis is usually present at the periphery of a cerebral abscess, infarct, hematoma, or metastatic cancer to the brain. The crushed brain tissue samples show loose clusters of atypical glial cells and loops of blood vessels without marginated glial cells (Fig. 13-2).

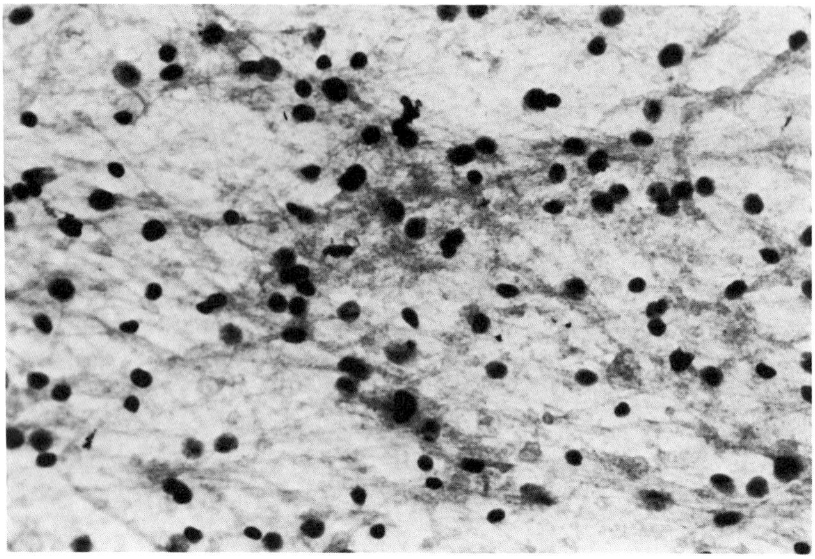

Figure 13-2. Reactive gliosis showing abundant atypical glial cells. (Hematoxylin and eosin ×250.)

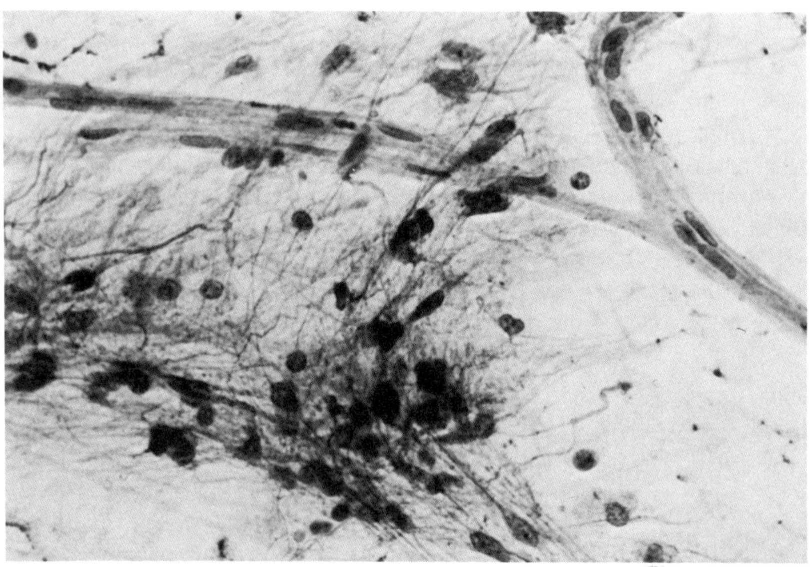

Figure 13-3. Low-grade astrocytoma. Branching thick-walled blood vessels with marginated astrocytes displaying slightly atypical nuclei. (Hematoxylin and eosin ×250.)

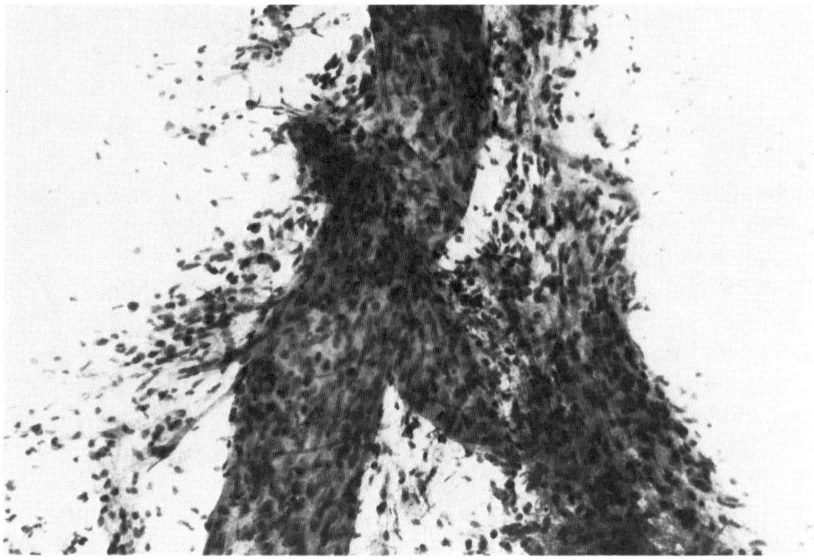

A

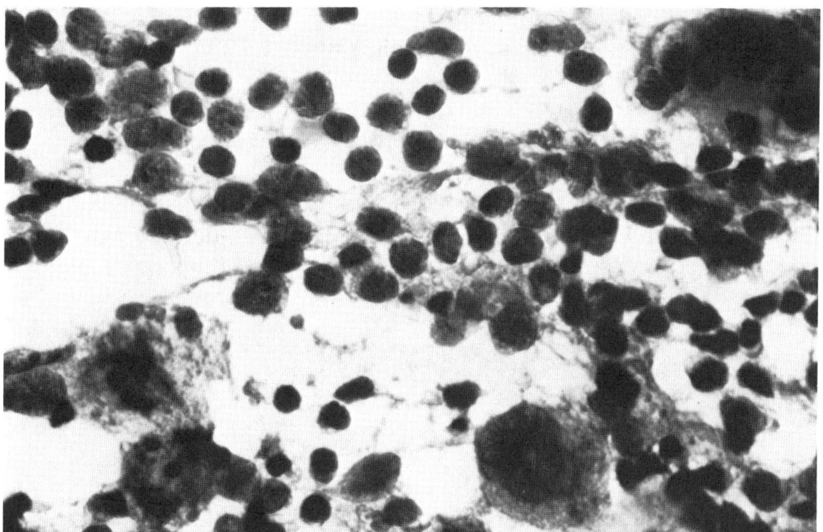

B

Figure 13-4. A. High-grade astrocytoma. Large blood vessels with marginated and pleomorphic tumor cells. **B.** High-grade astrocytoma showing pleomorphic tumor cells. (Hematoxylin and eosin **A.** ×100, **B.** ×400.)

TUMORS OF THE CEREBRUM AND CEREBELLUM

Neuroectodermal Tumors

Astrocytoma. Histologically, astrocytomas are usually classified into four grades (1 to 4). By ABC, however, they may be confidently classified into two groups of low-grade and high-grade tumors.

The cytodiagnosis of low-grade astrocytomas (grade 1 and 2 tumors) is difficult. Grade 1 tumor can not accurately be diagnosed by the crush preparation technique. Its cytologic pattern is similar to that of normal brain tissue or brain tissue with reactive gliosis. Grade 2 astrocytomas are characterized by the presence of a few thick-walled blood vessels surrounded by numerous benign-appearing or atypical astrocytes, which are randomly scattered in the smears or marginated around slightly thick-walled blood vessels (Fig. 13-3).

High-grade astrocytomas (grade 3 and 4 tumors) are easily identified in cytologic materials. They are characteristically hypercellular and rich in large fragments of thick-walled blood vessels surrounded by numerous pleomorphic tumor cells that vary in size and shape and display single or multiple large hyperchromatic nuclei (Fig. 13-4A and B). The gemistocytic variant astrocytoma belongs to the high-grade tumor group. It shows large pleomorphic malignant cells with abundant eosinophilic cytoplasm and eccentrically located nuclei (Fig. 13-5). Necrotic debris, inflammatory cells, and red blood cells are background substances.

Oligodendroglioma. The cytology of oligodendroglioma is usually characteristic. The cells possess uniformly oval or round nuclei and ill-defined cytoplasm with radial and wispy processes. They appear in monolayered rings surrounding empty round spaces (Fig. 13-6).

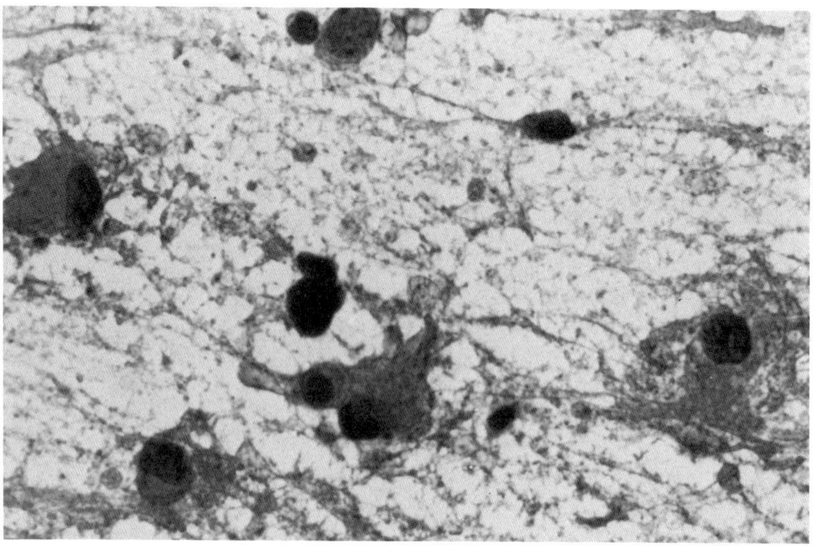

Figure 13-5. High-grade astrocytoma, gemistocytic type. (Hematoxylin and eosin ×400.)

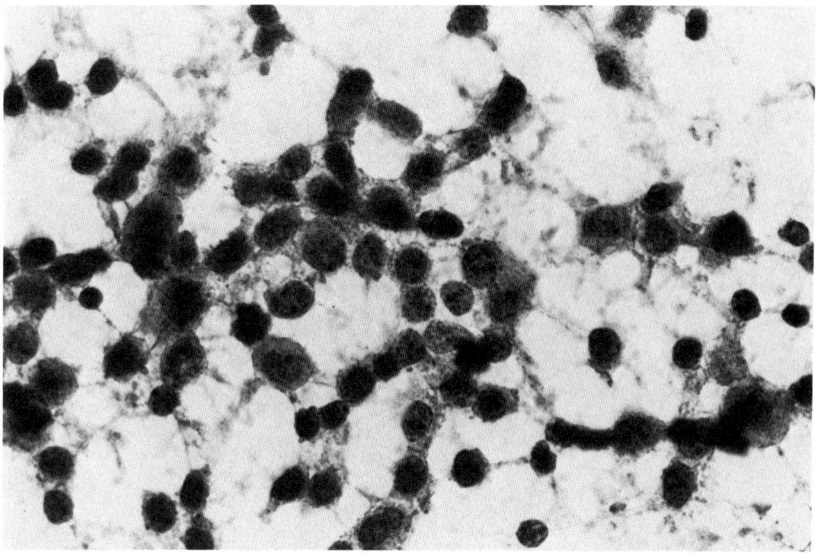

Figure 13-6. Oligodendroglioma. Single cells with wispy and ill-defined cytoplasm forming rings. (Hematoxylin and eosin ×400.)

Medulloblastoma. In crush preparations the small cells of a medulloblastoma occur singly or in dyshesive clusters. They show pleomorphic and hyperchromatic nuclei, and scanty cytoplasm (Fig. 13-7). They mimic those of a metastatic bronchogenic oat cell carcinoma. However, the midline location of the neoplasm in the cerebellum, the young age of the patient, and the absence of multifocal tumor masses are important features of a medulloblastoma.

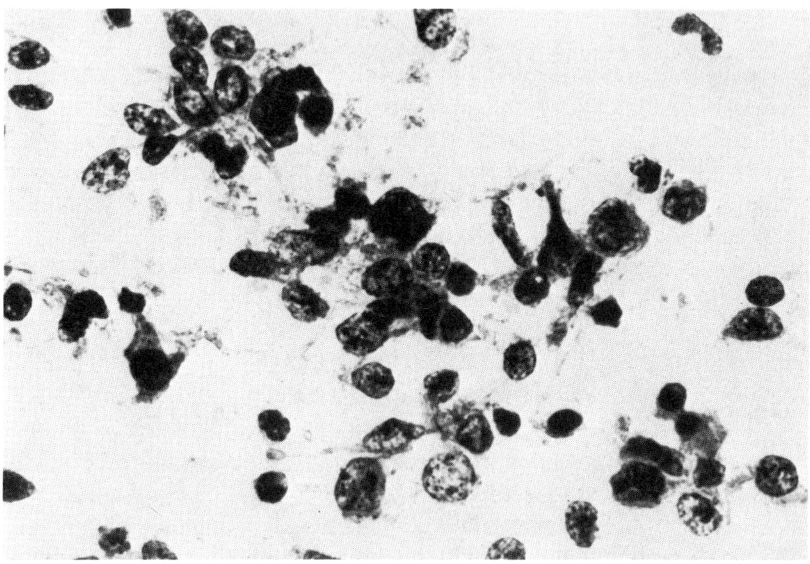

Figure 13-7. Medulloblastoma. Single and clustered small pleomorphic malignant cells with scant cytoplasm. (Hematoxylin and eosin ×400.)

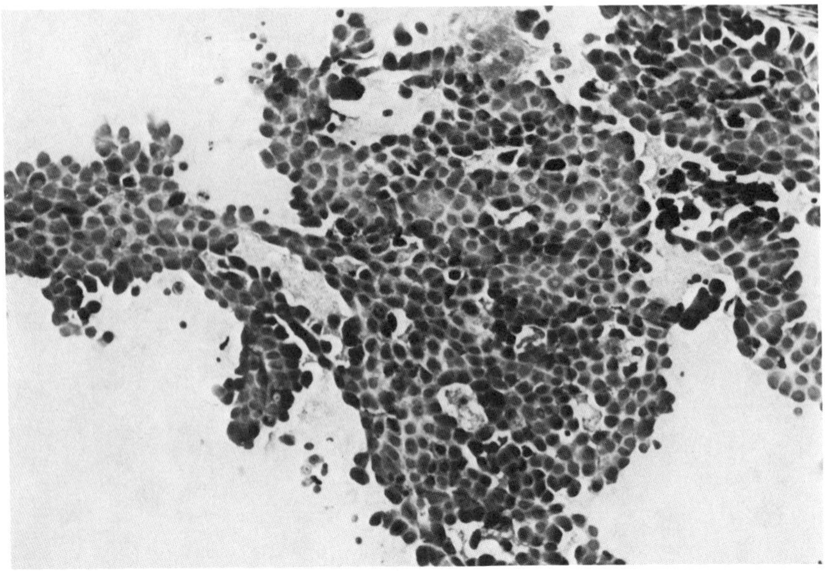

Figure 13-8. Ependymoma (epithelial type). Sheets of polygonal cells with round nuclei. (Hematoxylin and eosin ×100.)

Ependymoma. There are two histologic types of ependymomas. The epithelial type is usually seen in the cerebral hemisphere and posterior fossa. The papillary-type tumor, with or without myxomatous changes, usually occurs in the filum terminale of the spinal cord. The cells of cellular ependymomas are columnar or cuboidal and benign-appearing. They are present in irregular clusters or sheets (Fig. 13-8). Mucus-like material is readily identifiable in smears from tumors with myxomatous changes.

Choroid plexus papilloma and carcinoma. The choroid plexus papilloma has distinctive cytologic characteristics in crush preparations. It yields cells in three-dimensional clusters, showing round or oval nuclei with a finely granular chromatin pattern (Fig. 13-9). The rare carcinoma arising from the choroid plexus mimics a metastatic adenocarcinoma histologically. By means of ABC it displays small groups or isolated malignant glandular cells.

Cytologic features of neuroectodermal tumors of the brain are summarized in Table 13-1.

Metastatic Cancer

Metastatic carcinomas constitute less than 25% of all brain tumors, and they are usually multifocal. Of these neoplasms, bronchogenic carcinomas are the commonest, followed by breast carcinomas. Malignant melanoma is relatively common, and malignant lymphoma may involve the brain as part of its dissemination. Metastatic carcinomas from the kidney, colon, pancreas, prostate, and testis are rare. The cellular manifestations in crush or smear preparations are similar to those of the same tumor types in other sites of the body (see Chapters 6, 8–10, 12).

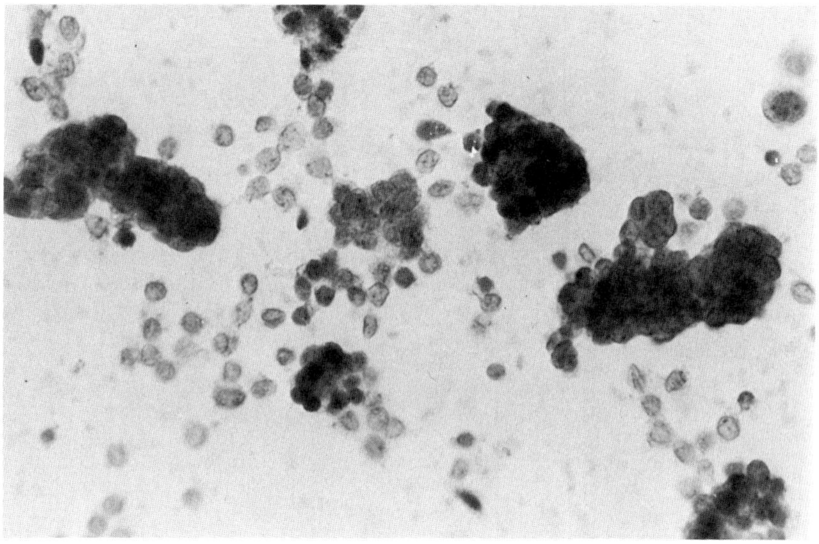

Figure 13-9. Choroid plexus papilloma. Tridimensional clusters of benign and regular tumor cells. (Hematoxylin and eosin ×250.)

PITUITARY ADENOMA

Pituitary adenomas occasionally expand upward above the sella turcica and appear as a deep-seated brain tumor. In these cases CT-guided needle biopsy is needed to secure tissue for diagnosis. The crush preparation shows cells with round nuclei, conspicuous nucleoli, and ill- or well-defined cytoplasm. They occur singly or in loose clusters. Intranuclear cytoplasmic inclusions may be seen (Fig. 13-10).

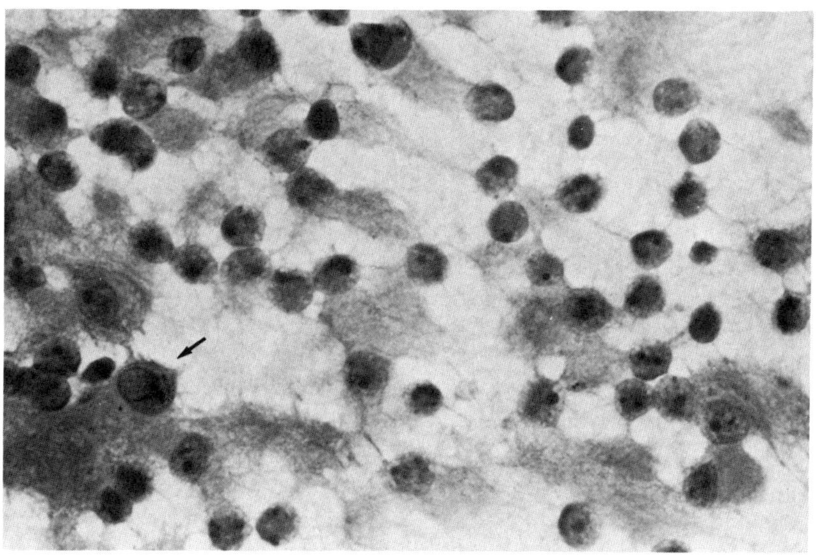

Figure 13-10. Pituitary adenoma. Single or clustered epithelial cells with ill-defined abundant cytoplasm and round nuclei with conspicuous nucleoli. An intranuclear cytoplasmic inclusion is noted (*arrow*). (Hematoxylin and eosin ×400.)

Table 13-1. Cytologic Features of Neuroectodermal Tumors of the Brain

CELLULAR CHARACTERISTICS	ASTROCYTOMA LOW-GRADE	ASTROCYTOMA HIGH-GRADE	OLIGODENDROGLIOMA	MEDULLOBLASTOMA	EPENDYMOMA
Cell arrangement	Tumor cells marginated around thin-wall vessels	Tumor cell aggregates, marginated around thick-wall vessels	Monolayered forming rings	Single and loosely grouped	Cohesive clusters or sheets
Tumor cells					
Appearance	Atypical astrocytes	Pleomorphic astrocytes with single or multiple nuclei	Monomorphic cells with round, hyperchromatic nuclei	Small, pleomorphic cells with hyperchromatic nuclei	Cuboidal or columnar cells with bland, oval nuclei
Cytoplasm	Scant	Variable Gemistocytic variant abundant, granular	Ill-defined	Scant	Well-defined
Blood vessel proliferation	++	+++	±	±	–

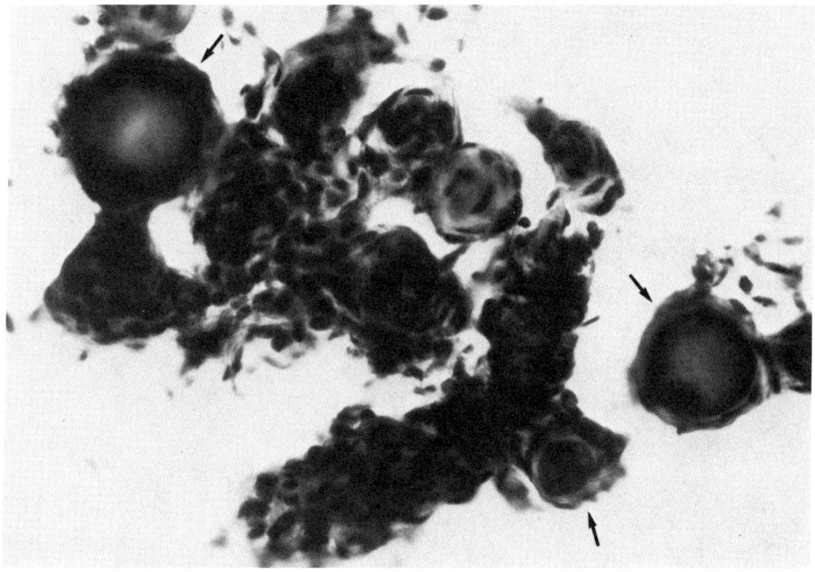

Figure 13-11. Psammomatous meningioma showing tight clusters of tumor cells in whorling pattern and psammoma bodies (*arrow*). (Hematoxylin and eosin ×250.)

MENINGIOMA

Meningioma and acoustic neuroma are rare targets of stereotactic CT-guided needle biopsy, because a preoperative diagnosis of these neoplasms usually is made by means of an imaging technique. In aberrant locations, however, these tumors may simulate a deep-seated glioma clinically or radiologically.

In general, meningioma tissue fragments are easy to crush and show little artefact. Both psammomatous- and meningotheliomatous-type meningiomas display characteristic features. Psammomatous tumor shows tight clusters of tumor cells arranged in papillary and whorled patterns. Individual tumor cells display round or oval nuclei and scanty ill-defined cytoplasm. Psammoma bodies are noted within cell clusters and in the smear background (Fig. 13-11). The meningotheliomatous meningioma shows tumor cells present mainly in small sheets or clusters. They have abundant, well-defined, filmy cytoplasm and round or oval nuclei having a finely granular chromatin pattern and small nucleoli (Fig. 13-12).

ACOUSTIC NEUROMA OR NEURILEMOMA

Tissue fragments from neurilemomas are hard and difficult to crush. Under low power, the crushed tissue presents as thick irregular fragments with sharp borders. In thin areas of tissue fragments the cells show ill-defined cytoplasm. Their nuclei are round, oval, or irregularly shaped and display a moderate degree of pleomorphism. Foamy histiocytes are present among the neoplastic cells. Tumor cells ar-

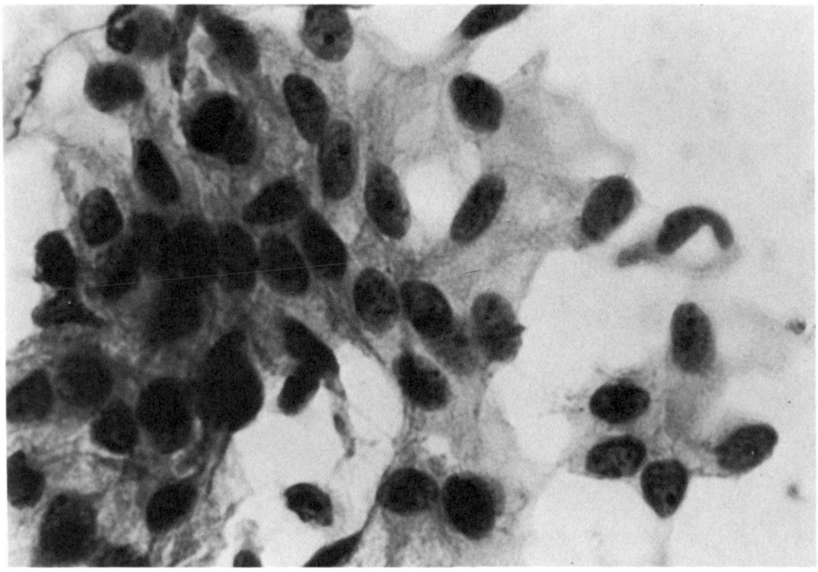

Figure 13-12. Meningotheliomatous meningioma showing sheets of tumor cells with thin cytoplasm. (Hematoxylin and eosin ×400.)

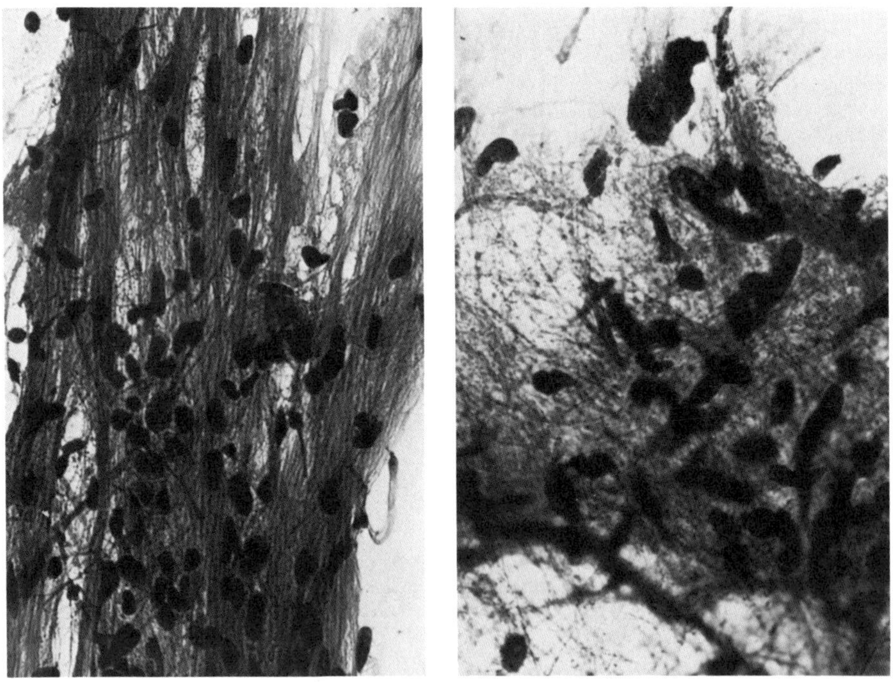

A B

Figure 13-13. A. Neurilemoma showing a bundle of tumor cells with fibrillary cytoplasm and somewhat atypical nuclei. (Hematoxylin and eosin ×400.) **B.** Ancient neurilemoma showing pleomorphic nuclei. (Hematoxylin and eosin ×400.)

Table 13-2. Comparative Cytomorphology of Meningiomas and Neurilemomas

CELLULAR CHARACTERISTICS	MENINGIOMA	NEURILEMOMA
Tumor tissue consistency	Soft, easy to crush	Hard, difficult to crush
Cell arrangement	Thin sheets, Small groups	Thick, large tissue fragments
Tumor cells		
Shape	Variable Polygonal Spindle	Pleomorphic
Cytoplasm	Well-defined	Ill-defined
Nuclei	Oval	Pleomorphic
Crushing artifacts	−	++
Psammoma bodies	±	−
Foamy histiocytes	−	++
Pyknotic tumor cell nuclei	−	++

ranged in pallisades are rarely observed (Fig. 13-13A). Crushed tissues from long-standing or ancient neurilemomas display bizarre nuclei, some of which are pyknotic (Fig. 13-13B).

Distinctive features of meningiomas and neurilemomas in crush preparations are summarized in Table 13-2.

DIAGNOSTIC ACCURACY AND PITFALLS

Cytodiagnosis of neuroectodermal tumors of the brain in most situations is not difficult. A diagnostic accuracy of over 90% may be expected with representative samples. Low-grade astrocytomas are difficult to be distinguished from reactive gliosis. Brain tissue from the Ammon's horn of the hippocampus may show bizarre cells mimicking those of a high-grade astrocytoma. Meningiomas and neurilemomas have distinctive cytologic features that are quite different from those of neuroectodermal tumors of the brain. Low-power view is very helpful in discriminating neurilemoma from meningioma. Both high-grade astrocytoma and long-standing neurilemoma show marked cellular pleomorphism, but blood vessels are not seen in smears from neurilemoma.

SUGGESTED READING

Chandrasoma PT, Apuzzo MLJ: *Stereotactic Brain Biopsy*. New York, Igaku-Shoin, 1989.

Daumas-Dupont C, Scheithauer BW, Kelly PJ: A histologic and cytologic method for the spatial definition of gliomas. Mayo Clin Proc 1987;62:435–449.

Mouriquand C, Benabid A, Breyton M: Stereotactic cytology of brain tumors. Review of an eight-year experience. *Acta Cytol* 1987;31:756–764.

Nguyen GK, Johnson ES, Mielke BW: Cytology of meningiomas and neurilemomas in crush preparations. A useful adjunct to frozen section diagnosis. *Acta Cytol* 1988;32:362–366.

Nguyen GK, Johnson ES, Mielke BW: Cytology of neuroectodermal tumors of the brain in crush preparations. A review of 56 cases of deep-seated tumors sampled by CT-guided stereotactic needle biopsy. *Acta Cytol* 1989;33:67–73.

Rubenstein LJ: Tumors of the central nervous system. In *Atlas of Tumor Pathology*, ed 2. Washington, DC, Armed Forces Institutes of Pathology, 1972.

Silverman JF: Cytopathology of fine-needle aspiration biopsy of the brain and spinal cord. *Diagn Cytopathol* 1986;2:312–319.

Willems JGMS, Alva-Willems JM: Accuracy of cytodiagnosis of central nervous system neoplasms in stereotactic biopsies. *Acta Cytol* 1984;28:243–249.

14

DNA QUANTITATION

In recent years, DNA quantitation has been performed more routinely on cell and tissue samples of malignant tumors to predict the prognosis of cancer patients. The DNA measurement may be done by means of cytophometry or flow cytometry. It has been documented that normal and benign cells are diploid or polydiploid, while malignant cells may be diploid, polydiploid or aneuploid. These important findings can be used to identify aneuploid malignant cells, especially when the cytomorphologic diagnosis is inconclusive. A brief review of the cell cycle is helpful for the interpretation of DNA histograms.

CELL CYCLE

A proliferating cell goes through different phases or gaps before mitosis. These phases are indicated as G1, S, G2, and M (Fig. 14-1).

The G1 phase occupies over one-half of the total cell generation life. During G1, only protein and RNA syntheses occur, and the cell does not synthesize DNA. S represents the DNA synthesis phase of the cell. At the beginning of the S phase, each diploid cell contains two copies of each chromosome (2N or 2C), and by the end of the phase its DNA content doubles (4N or 4C). G2 is the period of RNA and protein syntheses prior to mitosis. Cells in G2 and mitotic phase (M) can not be distinguished on the basis of DNA content, as their nuclear DNA distributions are similar (4N or 4C). The daughter cells produced by mitosis (M) are diploid (2N or 2C). They may continue through the cell cycle for further replication or enter into a resting state referred to as G0, where they may remain indefinitely or be recruited

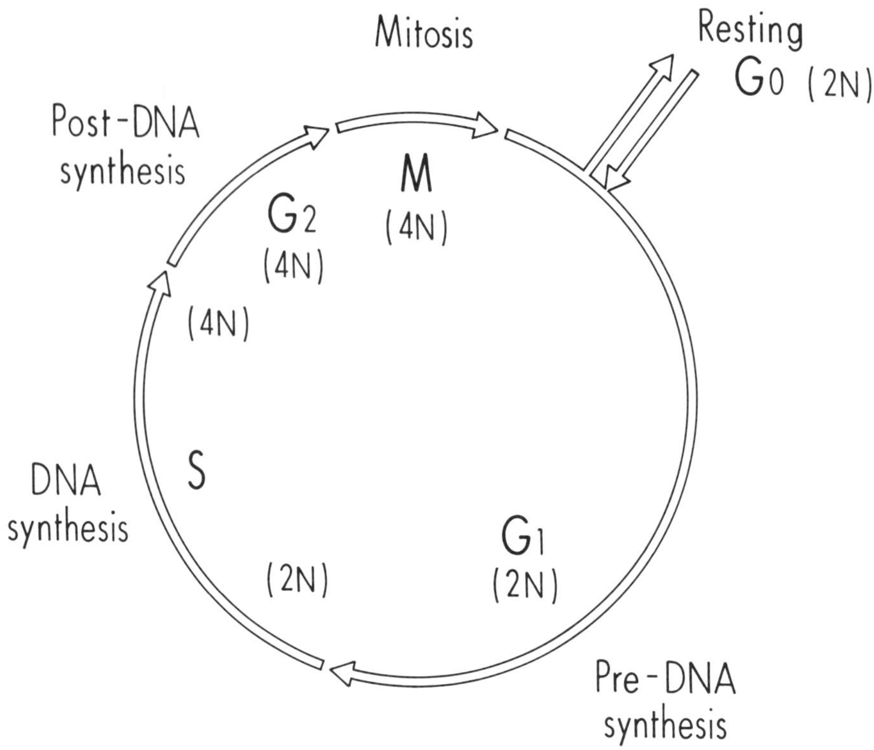

Figure 14-1. Cycle of a proliferating cell, showing different phases or gaps. DNA contents of the cell are shown within *brackets*.

back into the cycle. Cells in G1 and G0 contain a similar amount of DNA; thus, they are indistinguishable on the basis of DNA content.

DNA QUANTITATION METHODS

Cytophotometry. The DNA quantitation is carried out on a Feulgen- or acridine orange-stained smear. Usually, the measurement is performed randomly on 100 to 200 morphologically identified cells. The normal epithelial cells and lymphocytes present on the smear are used as an internal diploid standard for the determination of the modal value of the tumor cells studied on the histogram generated (Fig. 14-2A–C). The main advantage of this measurement method is the use of the same clinical sample for both routine cytomorphologic study and DNA quantitation. In other words, it permits the determination of DNA content-specific cell type. The disadvantages of cytophotometry include the bias of the observer in the subjective selection of cells for measurement, the small number of cells measured, and the time-consuming nature of the procedure. The presence of necrotic debris and cell secretory products such as mucous material may cause difficulties in DNA measurement.

Flow cytometry. This technique can determine the DNA content or ploidy of a large number of single cells or nuclei in a short period of time. The cells in suspension are stained with one of several fluorescent dyes that bind specifically and stoichiometrically to DNA. Propidium iodide and acridine orange are the most commonly used fluorochromes. Usually, normal lymphocytes, chicken red blood cells, or trout red blood cells, which are known to be diploid cells, are added to the test sample for the determination of the diploid standard. The histogram obtained shows several peaks. To determine the ploidy of the cells studied, the DNA index is calculated. This is done by dividing the G1/G0 DNA peak channel of the studied cells by the G1/G0 peak channel of the diploid standard cells. If the ratio is not equal to

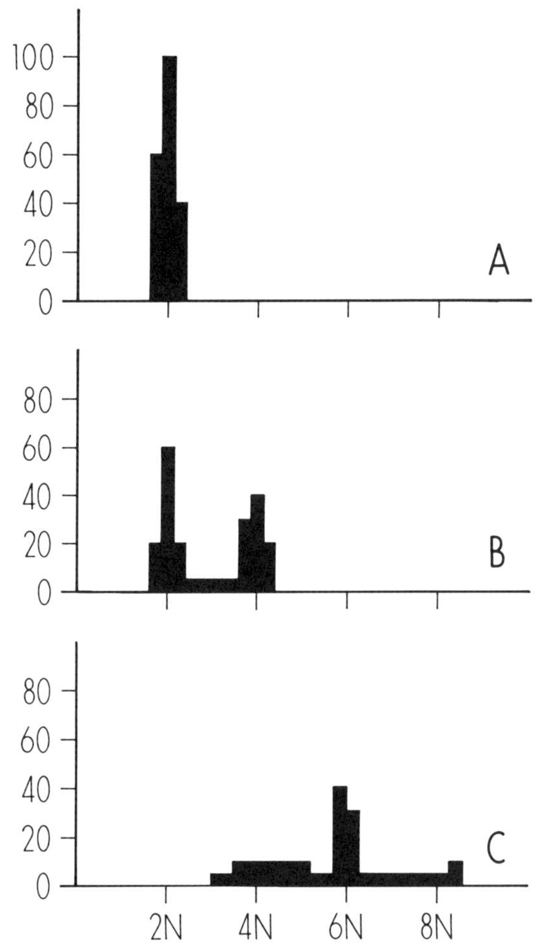

Figure 14-2. Cytophotometry histograms generated by DNA measurements of cancer cells. **A.** Diploid cancer cells showing a ploidy pattern similar to that of nongrowing, normal G0/G1 cells. **B.** Polydiploid cancer cells showing a DNA histogram similar to that of proliferating normal cells (G0/G1, S, G2/M cells). **C.** Aneuploid cancer cells showing a DNA histogram with marked variations from the norm.

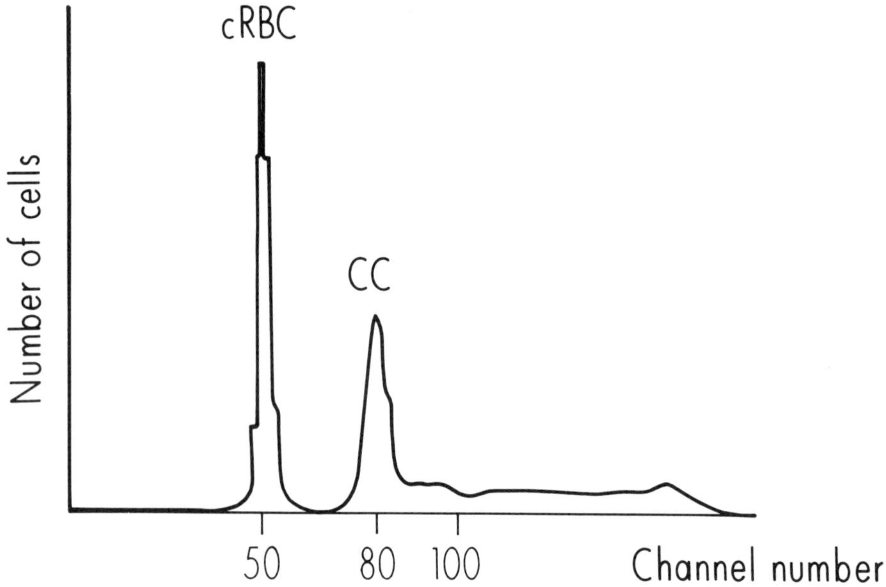

Figure 14-3. Flow cytometry histogram generated from DNA measurements of aneuploid cancer cells. Note the diploid peak of control chicken red blood cells (cRBC) at channel 50 and the aneuploid peak of the cancer cells (CC) at channel 80. The DNA index of the cancer cells is 1.6, indicating their aneuploid pattern.

1.0 the cells studied are aneuploid (Fig. 14-3). One of the main disadvantages of the flow cytometry is its inability to morphologically distinguish cancer cells from benign cells. For a pure tumor cell population, such as a cultured cell line, flow cytometry can determine its DNA content or ploidy with accuracy. However, clinical specimens usually contain heterogenous cell populations that lead to interpretive difficulties of flow cytometry histograms. In histograms of samples containing numerous benign cells and a small number of aneuploid cancer cells, the aneuploid peak of the latter may be totally masked by the predominant diploid peak of the former. Thus, ploidy determination by flow cytometry has a limited value in the detection of cancer cells in NAB samples.

SUGGESTED READING

Atkin B, Mattison G, Baker MC: Comparison of the DNA content and chromosome number of fifty human tumours. *Br J Cancer* 1966;20:87–101.

Auer G, Askensten U, Erharot K, et al.: Comparison between slide and flow cytophotometric DNA measurements in breast tumors. *Anal Quant Cytol Histol* 1987;9:138–146.

Johnson TS, Katz RL, Pershouse M: Flow cytometric application in cytopathology. *Anal Quant Cytol Histol* 1988;10:423–458.

Greenebaum E, Koss LG, Sherman AB, et al.: Comparison of needle aspiration and solid biopsy technics in the flow cytometric study of DNA distributions of surgically resected tumors. *Am J Clin Pathol* 1984;82:559–564.

Remvikos Y, Magdelenat H, Zajdela A: DNA flow cytometry applied to fine needle sampling of human breast cancer. *Cancer* 1988;61:1629–1634.

Rosen S, Mercer WE: Cytophotometry of breast carcinoma: acridin-orange DNA microfluorometry with Giemsa counterstain. *Anal Quant Cytol Histol* 1985;159–162.

Sanchez MA, Auer G, Zetterberg A: Advances in cytology. In Linsk JA, Franzen S: *Clinical Aspiration Cytology*. ed 2. Philadelphia, Lippincott, 1989, pp 421–434.

APPENDIX

QUESTIONS (ANSWERS p. 178)

Select the **single** best answer:

1) In experienced hands the diagnostic accuracy of breast cancers by ABC can reach:
   A—95%
   B—80%
   C—85%
   D—90%
   E—75%
2) The mean false-negative rate of cytodiagnosis of thyroid tumors by ABC is about:
   A— 9%
   B—15%
   C—20%
   D— 1%
   E— 5%
3) False-positive diagnosis of Hashimoto's disease is mainly due to the presence of:
   A—Abundant lymphocytes
   B—Hyperplastic follicular cells
   C—Hyperplastic Hürthle cells
   D—Lack of clinical information
   E—All of the above
4) ABC of an anaplastic carcinoma of the thyroid may mimic that of:
   A—Hürthle cell carcinoma
   B—Medullary carcinoma
   C—Thyroid abcess
   D—Colloid goiter with hemorrhagic degenerative change
   E—Colloid goiter with toxic nodule

5) A false-positive diagnosis of an adenolymphoma of the salivary gland may be due to:
A—Numerous oncocytes
B—Numerous lymphocytes
C—Degenerated oncocytes
D—Marked cystic degenerative changes
E—Marked lymphoid hyperplasia

6) Diagnostic accuracy rate of large-cell lymphoma by ABC is about:
A—40%
B—50%
C—60%
D—70%
E—90%

7) ABC of a well-differentiated lymphoma can be mistaken for that of a:
A—Reactive lymph node
B—Meckel cell tumor
C—Metastatic oat cell carcinoma
D—Eccrine poroma
E—None of the above

8) Bizarre cancer cells aspirated from a renal mass are most commonly originated from a:
A—Wilms' tumor
B—Sarcoma of the kidney
C—Sarcomatoid renal cell carcinoma
D—Xanthomatous pyelonephritis
E—Adrenal cortical carcinoma invading the kidney

9) Diagnostic accuracy rate of lung cancers by percutaneous NAB is about:
A—90%
B—80%
C—70%
D—60%
E—None of the above

10) The false-positive cytodiagnostic rate of NAB of the lung reported in the literature is as high as:
A—3%
B—8%
C—12%
D—15%
E—None of the above

11) Cells of a carcinoid tumor may mimic:
A—Hyperplastic reserve cells
B—Lymphocytes
C—Oat cell carcinoma cells
D—Cells of a small cell adenocarcinoma
E—All of the above

12) The most important cytochemical or immunocytochemical staining for the differential diagnosis between an adenocarcinoma and epitheliomatous malignant mesothelioma is:

A—PAS
B—Keratin and vimentin
C—CEA
D—Alcian blue
E—None of the above

13) Cytodiagnostic accuracy rate of pancreatic carcinoma by intraoperative NAB is about:
A—95%
B—85%
C—80%
D—75%
E—None of the above

14) False-positive cytodiagnosis of pancreatic ABC may be related to the presence of:
A—Liver cells
B—Bile duct cells
C—Hyperplastic endocrine cells
D—All of the above
E—None of the above

15) Cytoplasmic "pale bodies" are commonly seen in ABC of:
A—Fibrolamellar hepatocellular carcinoma
B—Poorly differentiated hepatocellular carcinoma
C—Well-differentiated hepatocellular carcinoma
D—Liver cell adenoma
E—Metastatic endoderneal sinus tumor to liver

16) Intracytoplasmic hyaline bodies are seen more commonly in ABC of a:
A—Well differentiated hepatocellular carcinoma
B—Poorly differentiated hepatocellular carcinoma
C—Liver cell adenoma
D—Nodular hyperplasia of the liver
E—Cholangiocarcinoma

17) Intranuclear cytoplasmic inclusions are seen in cells of:
A—Cirrhotic liver
B—Normal liver
C—Hepatocellular carcinoma
D—All of the above
E—None of the above

18) The most important test(s) for the differential diagnosis between a renal cell carcinoma and adrenal cortical carcinoma is(are):
A—Keratin and vimentin stainings
B—CEA
C—Ploidy determination by flow cytometry
D—Electron microscopic study of aspirated cells
E—None of the above

19) Blastematous cells of a Wilms' tumor mimic those of:
A—Lymphoma
B—Neuroblastoma
C—Round-cell sarcoma

D—All of the above
E—None of the above

20) Cells of the Ammon's horn of the hippocampus may mimic those of a:
A—Medulloblastoma
B—Metastatic adenocarcinoma
C—High-grade astrocytoma
D—Oligodendroglioma
E—Choroid plexus carcinoma

21) The presence of numerous foamy histiocytes is one of the characteristics in cell samples of:
A—Neurilemoma
B—Meningioma
C—High-grade astrocytoma
D—Metastatic malignant fibrous histiocytoma
E—All of the above

22) Which statement(s) is(are) true for cytophotometry:
A—It permits the determination of DNA content specific cell type
B—The procedure is time consumming
C—It suffers from the bias of the observer who selects the cells for measurement
D—All of the above
E—None of the above

23) Which statement(s) is(are) true for DNA quantitation by flow cytometry:
A—Interpretation of histogram of clinical material is difficult
B—Aneuploid peak of cancer cells may be masked by the diploid peak of benign cells present in the sample
C—Flow cytometry can not distinguish cancer cells from benign cells
D—All of the above
E—None of the above

24) The following is characteristic of pleomorphic adenoma:
A—Oxyphilic cells
B—Naked nuclei
C—Papillae
D—Isolated stellate cells
E—Lymphocytes

25) Intranuclear cytoplasmic inclusions are not associated with:
A—Melanoma
B—Hepatocytes
C—Pleomorphic adenoma
D—Papillary carcinoma of the thyroid
E—Medullary carcinoma of the thyroid

26) The most readily identified lymph node lesion by ABC is:
A—Hodgkin's disease
B—Poorly-differentiated lymphoma
C—Florid reactive hyperplasia
D—Well-differentiated lymphoma
E—Histiocytic lymphoma

27) Immunocytochemistry is least helpful in the definitive diagnosis of:

A—Metastatic bronchogenic carcinoma
B—Metastatic prostatic carcinoma
C—Metastatic follicular carcinoma
D—Metastatic melanoma
E—Metastatic medullary carcinoma

28) Most characteristic of the ABC from liposarcoma is:
A—Benign-appearing groups of fat cells
B—Myxomatous material
C—Round cells
D—Spindle cells
E—Lipoblasts

29) Spindle cell tumors of soft tissue are generally interpreted by:
A—The Papanicolaou stain
B—Positivity to Vimentin
C—Positivity to Demin
D—Multimodal approach
E—Identification of cigar-shaped nuclei

30) Cells of seminal vesicle origin do not show:
A—Triangular shape
B—Lipochrome pigment
C—Positivity to prostate specific antigen
D—Hyperchromatia
E—Large size

31) The ABC from papillary carcinoma of the breast does not usually show:
A—Papillae
B—Hemosiderin macrophage
C—Isolated cells
D—Cell paucity
E—Bland cells

For questions 32 through 60 select the best answer: #1—A,B,D,E; #2—A; #3—C,D; #4—A,B; #5—All

32) Characteristics of the ABC from oat cell carcinoma are:
A—Molding
B—Malignant diathesis
C—Vesicular nuclei
D—Scant cytoplasm
E—Hyperchromatic nuclei

33) The ABC of adenolymphoma of the salivary gland frequently shows:
A—Ghost cells
B—Lymphocytes
C—Naked nuclei
D—Spindle cells
E—Glandular cells

34) ABC criteria of malignancy most important to diagnosis include:
A—Dyshesion
B—Macronucleoli
C—Hyperchromasia
D—Cellularity
E—Nuclear membrane irregularity and thickening

35) A cell-poor aspirate may be due to:
A—Poor technique
B—Scar tissue
C—Chemotherapy
D—Radiation
E—Certain benign conditions
36) The ABC of neurogenic sarcoma shows:
A—Single cells with elongated nuclei
B—Biphasic cellular pattern
C—Vacuolated cytoplasm
D—Laminin negative
E—Scanty basal laminae
37) The ABC of fibrosarcoma shows:
A—Scanty rough endoplasmic reticulum
B—Smooth nuclear contour (EM)
C—Single and clustered spindled cells
D—Vimentin positive cytoplasm
E—Desmin positive cytoplasm
38) The ABC of angiosarcoma shows:
A—Rod-shaped tubular bodies (EM)
B—Loosely clustered cells
C—Thick tissue fragments
D—Numerous macrophages
E—Desmin positive cytoplasm
39) The ABC of spindle-cell melanoma shows:
A—Pinocytotic vesicles along cell membrane
B—Redundant basal laminae (EM)
C—Single cells
D—Macronucleoli
E—Abundant smooth endoplasmic reticulum
40) The ABC of pleomorphic malignant melanoma shows:
A—Two or three distinct cell populations
B—Intranuclear cytoplasmic inclusions
C—Clustered cells
D—Pinocytotic vesicles along cell membrane (EM)
E—Redundant basal laminae
41) The ABC of pleomorphic rhabdomyosarcoma shows:
A—Alpha-fetoprotein positivity
B—Vacuolated cytoplasm
C—Intracytoplasmic cross-striations, rare
D—Abundant, granular cytoplasm
E—None of the above
42) The ABC of lobular carcinoma of the breast shows:
A—Markedly irregular nuclei
B—Numerous lymphocytes
C—Cells in Indian filing
D—Intracytoplasmic mucous globules
E—Numerous hemosiderin laden macrophages
43) The ABC of renal oncocytoma shows:

A—Single, polygonal cells with granular cytoplasm
B—Inconspicuous nucleoli
C—Sheets of tumor cells
D—Macronucleoli
E—Abundant naked nuclei

44) The ABC of renal cell carcinoma shows:
A—Abundant smooth endoplasmic reticulum (EM)
B—Vimentin negative cytoplasm
C—Macronucleoli in high-grade tumor
D—Small groups or sheets of tumor cells
E—No naked nuclei

45) The ABC of subacute thyroiditis shows:
A—Abundant monomorphic lymphocytes
B—Scant follicular cells
C—Rare small multinucleated giant cells
D—Fibroblastic cells
E—Abundant colloid

46) The ABC of a papillary carcinoma of the thyroid shows:
A—Lymphoid cells, rare
B—Scant colloid
C—Cells mainly in dyshesive clusters
D—Psammoma bodies, rare
E—Nuclear grooves

47) The ABC of adenoid cystic carcinoma of the salivary glands shows:
A—Mucous cells
B—Squamous cells
C—Balls of basaloid cells
D—No lymphocytes
E—Papillae

48) The ABC of pleomorphic adenoma of the salivary gland shows:
A—Epithelial cell clusters
B—Mucoid material
C—Numerous naked nuclei
D—Oncocytes in syncytia
E—Hemorrhagic cystic contents

49) The ABC of branchial cleft cyst shows:
A—Atypical squamous cells
B—Neutrophils
C—Mucous cells
D—Follicular thyroid cells
E—Psammoma bodies

50) Which statement(s) is (are) correct for a carotid body tumor:
A—Well-defined cytoplasm
B—Cystic changes, common
C—Round cells, singly and in clusters
D—NSE positive cytoplasm
E—NAB is usually not contraindicated

51) The ABC of an astrocytoma shows:

A—Easily identifiable cells of the gemistocytic variant
B—Margination of tumor cells around vessels
C—Cells in cohesive clusters
D—Thin-walled vessels in low-grade tumor
E—Distinction between a reactive gliosis and a low grade tumor is difficult

52) The ABC of adrenal cortical carcinoma shows:
A—Naked tumor cell nuclei, rare
B—Vimentin negative tumor cells
C—Cells similar to those of renal cell carcinoma
D—Cells containing abundant smooth endoplasmic reticulum
E—Keratin negative tumor cells

53) The ABC of neuroendocrine tumor of the pancreas shows:
A—Cells, often seen singly
B—NSE positive
C—Syncytial tumor cell clusters not present
D—Vimentin, negative or positive
E—All of the above

54) The ABC of bronchioloalveolar cell carcinoma shows:
A—Mucus may be absent
B—Cells in cohesive large sheets
C—Macronucleoli, often multiple
D—Macronucleoli, rarely multiple
E—Nuclear chromatin may be bland

55) The ABC of large cell anaplastic carcinoma of the lung commonly shows:
A—Cells, singly and in loose aggregates
B—Macronucleoli, common
C—Cells in cohesive sheets
D—Nuclear molding
E—Abundant necrotic debris

56) The ABC of bronchogenic squamous carcinoma shows:
A—Macronucleoli, common
B—Fine chromatin pattern
C—Keratinized tumor cells, often singly
D—Non-keratinized tumor cells, often in syncytia
E—Necrotic debris, usually scant

57) Which statement(s) is(are) correct for ABC of prostatic adenocarcinoma:
A—Microglandular complexes, common in well-differentiated cancer
B—Loss of honeycomb pattern of tumor epithelium
C—Macronucleoli, common in well-differentiated tumor
D—Aspirates are often scant
E—Single cells, common in moderately differentiated cancer

58) ABC of benign prostatic enlargement commonly shows:
A—Scanty aspirate
B—Macronucleoli absent
C—Epithelial fragments with a vague honeycomb pattern
D—Microglandular complexes
E—Cellular crowding and piling

59) ABC of a hyperplastic lymph node shows:

A—Polymorphic lymphoid cell population
B—Tingible bodies in macrophages
C—Lymphoid cells with nuclear indentation
D—Lymphoid cells with nuclear protrusion
E—Necrotic debris, abundant

60) Differential cytologic features between cells from an adenocarcinoma and cells from a malignant mesothelioma include:
A—CEA positivity with adenocarcinoma cells
B—High molecular weight keratin positivity with mesothelioma cells
C—High molecular weight keratin positive for both tumors
D—CEA negativity with mesothelioma cells
E—Mucicarmine negativity with mesothelioma cells

ANSWERS

1	A	31	D
2	A	32	1
3	C	33	4
4	C	34	1
5	C	35	1
6	E	36	2
7	A	37	3
8	C	38	4
9	A	39	3
10	A	40	4
11	E	41	3
12	C	42	3
13	A	43	4
14	C	44	3
15	A	45	4
16	B	46	1
17	D	47	3
18	D	48	4
19	D	49	4
20	C	50	3
21	A	51	1
22	D	52	3
23	D	53	4
24	D	54	1
25	C	55	4
26	E	56	3
27	A	57	4
28	E	58	4
29	D	59	4
30	C	60	1

Index

A

Abcess
  liver, 129
  lung, 99
Acinic cell carcinoma, 48
Adenocarcinoma, *see specific organ*
Adenoid cystic carcinoma, salivary gland, 47
Adenolymphoma, 46
Adenoma, *see specific organ*
Adrenal, 146–151
  ABC, accuracy, 151
  ABC, indications, 139
  ABC, pitfalls, 151
  cortical adenoma, 146
  cortical carcinoma, 146
  metastatic cancer, 149
  pheochromocytoma, 146
Alpha fetoprotein, *see* Stains, immunocytochemical methods
Alveolar carcinoma, *see* Bronchioloalveolar cell carcinoma
Amoebic abcess, 129
Amyloid, 37
Anaplastic carcinoma, *see specific organ*
Ancient neurilemoma, 80, 163
Angioma, 81, 82
Angiomyolipoma, 141
Angiosarcoma, 81, 82
Apudoma, *see* Neuroendocrine tumor, metastatic pancreas
Aspergillosis, 102
Aspiration Biopsy Cytology (ABC), diagnostic criteria, diagnostic pitfalls, *see specific organs*
Astrocytoma, 156

B

Biopsy
  procedure, 7–9
  safety, 2
  utilization, *see specific organs*
Blastomycosis, 101–102
Bone, 72–77
  ABC, accuracy, 77
  ABC, indications, 72
  ABC, pitfalls, 77
  chondrosarcoma, 73
  chordoma, 73
  Ewing's sarcoma, 73
  giant cell tumor, 73
  metastatic cancers, 75–77
  multiple myeloma, 74
  osteogenic sarcoma, 73
Breast, 14–26
  ABC, accuracy, 26
  ABC, indications, 14
  ABC, pitfalls, 26
  apocrine cyst, *see* Breast, fibrocystic changes
  carcinoma, 20–25

Breast, carcinoma (*contd.*)
apocrine cell, 21
ductal, 20
lobular, 23
medullary, 20
mucinous, 20
papillary, 22
cyst, *see* Breast, fibrocystic changes
cystosarcoma phylloides, 18
ductal epithelial hyperplasia, 17
fat necrosis, 15
fibroadenoma, 18
fibrocystic changes, 15–17
mastitis, 14, 15
papilloma, 18
sarcoma, 26
subareolar papillomatosis, 18
Bronchioloalveolar cell carcinoma, 106
Bronchogenic carcinoma, *see* Lung

C
Calcitonin, *see* Stains, immunocytochemical methods
Candida, 104
Carcinoembryonic antigen, *see* Stains, immunocytochemical methods
Carcinoid tumor, lung, 111
Carotid body tumor, 50
Cholangiocarcinoma, 134
Chondrosarcoma, 73
Chordoma, 73
Choriocarcinoma, 67
Cirrhosis, 138
Coccidioidomycosis, 104
Colloid material, thyroid, 33
Colloid carcinoma, breast, *see* Mucinous carcinoma, breast
Colonic adenocarcinoma, 62
Complications of NAB, *see specific organ*
Computed tomography (CT) guided NAB, 9
Cystosarcoma phylloides, 18
Cyst, *see specific organ*

D
Dermoid cyst, *see* Teratoma
Diagnostic accuracy, *see specific organ*
Diagnostic criteria, *see specific organ*
Diagnostic pitfalls, *see specific organ*

E
Echinococcal cyst, *see* Hydatid cyst
Electron microscopic study, 11
Endothelium, 99
Ependymoma, 158
Epidermal inclusion cyst, 68
Epithelial membrane antigen, *see* Stains, immunocytochemical methods
Epithelioid sarcoma, 84
Equipment, NAB, 7, 8
Ewing's sarcoma, 73, 86

F
False negative diagnosis, *see specific organ*
False positive diagnosis, *see specific organ*
Fat necrosis, 15
Fibroadenoma, breast, 18
Fibroma, 79
Fibrosarcoma, 79
Fibrohistiocytomas, 81, 82
Follicular tumor, *see* Thyroid
Fungal infection, *see* Lung

G
Gallbladder carcinoma, 136
Ganglioneuroblastoma, 149
Ganglioneuroma, 149
Germ cell tumor, 64–67, 115
Giant cell carcinoma, lung, 109
Giant cell tumor, bone, 73
Goiter, *see* Thyroid

H
Hamartoma, 102
Hashimoto's disease, 30
Hemangioma, *see* Angioma
Hepatocellular carcinoma, 131–135
Histiocytic lymphoma, *see* Lymph node, lymphoma
Histoplasmosis, 104
Hodgkin's disease, 56

Hürthle cell tumor, 34
Hydatid cyst, 101
Hyperplasia
  lymphoid tissue, 55
  prostate, 89
Hyperthyroidism, 30

I

Immunocytochemistry, 12
  alpha fetoprotein, 12
  beta human chorionic gonadotropin, 12
  calcitonin, 12, 35
  carcinoembryonic antigen, 12
  desmin, 12, 82
  epithelial membrane antigen, 12
  factor VIII–related antigen, 12
  keratin, 12
  leukocyte common antigen, 12
  myoglobin, 12
  neuron-specific enolase, 12
  prostatic acid phosphatase, 12, 95
  prostate-specific antigen, 12, 95
  S-100 protein, 12, 67, 84
  thyroglobulin, 12
Indications for NAB, *see specific organ*
Infectious mononucleosis, 69
Inflammation, *see specific organ*
Intracytoplasmic pale bodies, 131
Intranuclear cytoplasmic inclusions
  anaplastic carcinoma, thyroid, 39
  follicular tumors, 32, 39
  hepatocellular carcinoma, 131
  Hürthle cell tumor, 39
  medullary carcinoma, 39
  papillary carcinoma, 32, 35, 39
  pituitary adenoma, 159
  regenerative hepatocyte, 137
Islet cell tumor, *see* Pancreas, neuroendocrine tumor

K

Kidney, 139–151
  ABC, accuracy, 151
  ABC, indications, 139
  ABC, pitfalls, 151
  angiomyolipoma, 141
  cyst, 140
  oncocytoma, 142
  renal cell carcinoma, 142–144
  Wilms' tumor, 144

L

Laboratory procedures, 7–13
Langerhans giant cell, 56, 100
Leiomyoma, 79
Leiomyosarcoma, 79
Lipoblast, 79
Lipoma, 77
Liposarcoma, 78, 79
Liver, 127–138
  ABC, accuracy, 138
  ABC, indications, 127
  ABC, pitfalls, 138
  abcess, 129
  adenoma, 129
  bile canaliculi, 128
  bile duct epithelium, 128
  carcinoma, cholangio, 134, 135
  carcinoma, hepatocellular, 131–135
  carcinoma, metastatic, 135, 136
  cirrhosis, 138
  cyst, non-parasitic, 129
  endothelium, 128
  hemangioma, 131
  hepatocytes, 128
  hydatid cyst, 129
  hyperplasia, 129
Lobular carcinoma, *see* Breast
Lung, 97–113
  ABC, accuracy, 112
  ABC, indications, 97
  ABC, pitfalls, 112
  abcess, 99
  bronchial adenoma, 111
  carcinoid tumor, 111
  carcinoma, bronchogenic, 105–110
    adenocarcinoma, 105
    bronchioloalveolar cell, 106
    large cell anaplastic, 107
    small cell anaplastic, 108
    squamous cell, 105
  carcinoma, metastatic, 111
  fungal infections, 101–104
    aspergillus, 104

Lung, fungal infections (*contd.*)
blastomyces, 104
candida, 104
coccidioides, 104
cryptococcus, 104
Mucor, 104
hamartoma, 102
hydatid cyst, 100
mesothelial cells, benign, 99
mesothelioma, 113
NAB, complications, 10
NAB, techniques, 9, 97, 98
pneumocystis carinii pneumonia, 99
tuberculoma, 99
Lymph node, 54–71
ABC, accuracy, 67–70
ABC, indications, 54
ABC, pitfalls, 69
hyperplasia, 55
infectious mononucleosis, 69
lymphadenitis, non-specific, 55
sarcoidosis, 55, 56
tuberculosis, 56
lymphoma, 56–59
Hodgkin's disease, 56
non-Hodgkin's, 56
metastatic cancer, 57–67
toxoplasmosis, 70

M

Mastitis, 14, 15
Mediastinum, 114–116
cysts, 114
germ cell tumors, 115
neural tumors, 115
thymoma, 115
Medullary carcinoma
breast, 20
thyroid, 35
Medulloblastoma, 157
Melanoma, 67
Meningioma, 161
Mesothelioma, 113
Metastatic cancer, *see specific organ*
Mucinous carcinoma, breast, 20
Mucoepidermoid carcinoma, salivary gland, 47
Mucormycosis, 102
Multiple myeloma, 74

N

Needles, biopsy, 7, 8
Neurilemoma, 79, 80, 161
Neuroblastoma, 86
Neuroendocrine tumor, metastatic, pancreas, 124
Neurofibroma, 81
Neuron-specific enolase, *see* Stains, immunocytochemical methods
Nuclear grooves, 32

O

Oat cell carcinoma, *see* Lung, carcinoma, bronchogenic, small cell anaplastic
Oncocytoma
kidney, 142
salivary gland, 46
Osteogenic sarcoma, 73

P

Pancreas, 117–126
ABC, accuracy, 24
ABC, indications, 117
ABC, pitfalls, 125
carcinoma
ampullary, 123
ductal, 121–123
metastatic, 123
mucinous cystic lesion, 121
neuroendocrine tumor, 124
pancreatitis, 119
pseudocyst, 120
Papillary carcinoma
breast, 22
thyroid, 32
Papillary cystadenoma lymphomatosum, *see* Adenolymphoma
Papilloma, *see* Breast
Parathyroid
adenoma, 41
carcinoma, 41
cyst, 41
Parotid gland, *see* Salivary glands
Pheochromocytoma, 146, 147
Physaliferous cells, *see* Chordoma
Pleomorphic adenoma, 145

Pleomorphic mesenchymal tumors, 81–86
Pneumocystis carinii pneumonia, 99
Pneumothorax as complication of NAB, 10
Prostate, 88–96
  ABC, accuracy, 94
  ABC, indications, 88
  ABC, pitfalls, 94, 95
  benign enlargement, 89
  carcinoma, 90–93
  prostatitis, 89
Prostatitis, *see* Prostate
Psammoma bodies
  meningioma, 161
  papillary carcinoma, thyroid, 32

R

Rectal cells, benign, 95
Reed-Sternberg cells, 56, 57
Renal cell carcinoma vs. adrenal cortical carcinoma, 151
Renal cells, normal, 140
Renal pelvis, carcinoma, 144, 145
Riedel's struma, 30
Round cell mesenchymal tumors, 86

S

Salivary glands, 43–53
  ABC, accuracy, 51
  ABC, indications, 43
  ABC, pitfalls, 51
  adenolymphoma, 46
  benign lymphoepithelial lesion, 45
  carcinoma
    acinic cell, 48
    adenoid cystic, 47
    in pleomorphic adenoma, 49
    metastatic, 49
    mucoepidermoid, 47
    squamous cell, 49
    undifferentiated, 49
  mixed tumor, *see* Pleomorphic adenoma
  papillary cystadenoma lymphomatosum, *see* Adenolymphoma
  pleomorphic adenoma, 45
  sialadenitis, 44
  Warthin's tumor, *see* Adenolymphoma
Sarcoidosis, 55
Schwannoma, *see* Neurilemoma
Sclerosing adenosis, *see* Breast, fibrocystic changes
Seeding of tumor cells, *see* Biopsy, safety
Seminal vesicle cells, 95
Seminoma, 64
Sialadenitis, 44
Soft tissue tumors, 77–86
  ABC, accuracy, 85
  ABC, indications, 77
  ABC, pitfalls, 85
  lipomatous tumors, 77–79
  metastatic cancer, 85
  pleomorphic tumors, 81, 83, 84
    epithelioid sarcoma, 84
    fibrous histiocytoma, 84
    leiomyosarcoma, high grade, 84
    pleomorphic liposarcoma, 84
    pleomorphic rhabdomyosarcoma, 84
    synovial sarcoma, biphasic, 84
  round-cell tumors, 82, 85–86
    Ewing's sarcoma, extraskeletal, 86
    embryonal rhabdomyosarcoma, 86
    neuroblastoma, 86
    round-cell liposarcoma, 86
  spindle-cell tumors, 79, 82
    angiomatous, 82
    fibromatous, 82
    leiomyomatous, 82
    neurogenic tumors, 82
Squamous cell carcinoma, *see also specific organ*
  diagnostic pitfalls, 69
Stains
  immunocytochemical methods, 12
  routine, 11
Synovial sarcoma, 84

T

Team approach, 3
Technique, aspiration biopsy, *see* Biopsy, procedure; *specific organ*
Teratoma, 65, 115
Thymoma, 115

Thyroglossal duct cyst, 28
Thyroid, 27–42
  ABC, accuracy, 38
  ABC, indications, 27
  ABC, pitfalls, 40
  carcinoma
    anaplastic, 37
    in children, 37
    follicular, 31
    medullary, 35
    metastatic, 37
    papillary, 32
  colloid nodule, 31
  cyst, 28
  follicular neoplasms, 31, 32
  Graves' disease, 30
  Hashimoto's disease, 30
  Hürthle cell tumor, 34
  lymphoma, 37
  thyroiditis, 28–30
Tingible macrophages, 55
Toxoplasmosis, 69
Transitional cell carcinoma, 63
Tuberculosis
  lung, 99
  lymph node, 55

U

Ultrasound (US) guided NAB, 9

V

Vascular tumor, *see* Liver; Soft tissue tumors

W

Warthin's tumor, *see* Adenolymphoma
Wilms' tumor, 144